Lose Fat
By
Reducing Stress

By

Esther Lehman

Maale Adumim, Israel

ISBN-13: 978-1499580310

Published by Lose Fat Club

At CreateSpace

June 24th 2014

Esther Lehman

Maale Adumim, Israel

https://holylandoils.com

Printed in the United States of America

Table of Contents

INTRODUCTION

Start losing weight TODAY!!!

You woke up this morning and looked in the mirror as you have done every morning for the last number of years, and like every one of those mornings you get depressed by what you see. If only your reflection would show you a better and thinner you, God knows how hard you try. You have been on every diet fad out on the internet that promises you magical success in the fastest time. Under the circumstances who can blame you for raising your hopes "maybe this time next week I will have lost 20lbs," and when that doesn't happen you cannot help hating the way you look even more. Wishing away your fat stomach, large thighs, flabby arms and thick legs, is not going to make you lose that fat any faster, and this makes you feel completely helpless.

Searching for magic potions to transform your body into perfection, is what most people who suffer from obesity do. However, to get rid of your fat and reduce your circumference forever, to match that inner image you yearn for your body to be to make you happy, you need to have an action plan.

Women in general have a much harder time losing weight and I would say you have many valid reasons for certain types of weight gain. I recognize and acknowledge this first as a woman myself, and second because this is my profession. I know there is nothing scarier than the feeling of losing control of your body. It probably feels to you that your body seems to have a mind of its own, growing fatter, changing its shape and size as it chooses.

It must be so maddening that no matter what you do, and I know you've tried everything, each time you look in the mirror or get on the scales to weigh yourself, you see that you have gained yet more weight. This is the panic point, you scream internally, you lose hope and have no idea what else you should try.

It gets even more frustrating when you get seemingly friendly "advice" from well-meaning concerned friends, who notice every ounce you gain. You would like to strangle your partner or the next person in your family who mentions your weight. They don't understand you or have compassion to see your suffering. They don't get why you fret about your weight; they do not believe you when you claim that you eat healthily and exercise regularly. Deep down you hear them thinking "if you do everything right, how are you Fat!!!

I believe you; I really do...I know you have tried every diet, read every article, bought every product promising you miracles, and spent a lot of money, heartache and tears on this issue. You would not be reading this book had you not tried everything under the sun.

What is really keeping your body fat? Well, it could be one of three things or all three.

Number One, your body is most likely to be in what is called stress mode or may also be called survival mode.

Second Possibility is that your body is set itself into its safe mode.

The Third reason is that you may have a medical problem lurking, like an underactive thyroid, diabetes, or gastrointestinal inflammations such as an undiagnosed celiac disease.

Blood tests are always a good indication to see what is going on internally so that nutrition and natural treatments will be able to help. I recommend that you ask your doctor to send you for general blood tests including vitamin B12, folic acid, thyroid, sugar levels, vitamin D, LDL cholesterol, HDL, triglycerides, and liver function.

Chapter 1

Weight Loss Mindset

Acknowledge that your body is not listening to you.

How many times have you heard friends say that they want to lose 50lbs, in two weeks for a relatives' wedding? Then they proceed to starve themselves for those two weeks and lose a few pounds. Even though they never got to their original goal, they view their weight loss as a success. Until they realize that is was actually a failure when they see their bodies drastic reaction to this abuse.

These diets set your bodies up for failure, realistic goals mean losing weight slowly with methodical patience as part of a healthy lifestyle plan. Feeling a failure is most likely to trigger a food binge causing the person to regain back all their lost weight and more.

Starvation behaviour also forces your body to store food as fat, remember your bodies are a very smart and logical machine. You are comprised of many systems that work in harmony with each other, each relying on the other to do their tasks. Your body metabolism understands regularity, when food does not arrive as expected your body is forced to use itself as a food source.

This is not good, since your body will take its nutritional sources from your own stored proteins and collagen. Your bodies need energy to survive and eating irregularly forces your body to learn that it must store any food you eat as fat. Now you have developed a problem that will make it harder or even almost impossible for you to lose weight any time in the near future.

You can solve this situation, even though it is not a magical solution and involves you being disciplined and structured. You must start re-teaching your body to learn to trust you again, this is the only way that it will stop your bodies being in survival mode. For some people, it can take months for others it may take years of eating regularly. This depends on how long a person have abused your bodies for, but it can be done.

Chapter 2

Your SELF Perception

What does your internal mirror reflect externally?

Let's put talking about nutrition aside for now. Nutrition is a huge factor you should be taking into consideration, but now let's talk about how you feel towards yourself. Feeling good about yourselves reflects strongly upon the way you look and act, and people respond to you accordingly. Speaking nicely to yourselves sets a whole different image out there, than if you are convincing yourselves and hence others, that you are ugly and fat. Not only is this unproductive, it is detrimental to your subconscious mind and this literally gives others a license to treat you with the same disrespect that you give yourself.

The danger of this is reducing yourself to allowing others to control your confidence. Why should you let others have the chance to slip inside your inner self perception, and thus feed your subconscious mind with untrue information and shake your self-confidence? Having a bad body image while anticipating achieving the perfect body is completely contradictory. These thoughts process cannot connect since they are two different extremes. Negative emotions are so strong and powerful, it is as though you are wishing and willing fervently for what you don't want.

As a Naturopath, I believe your physical self and your emotional self are connected. For example, when you feel nervous or happy, angry or sad, these are strong emotions that your body feels physically. These feelings are generated by your thoughts that cause this powerful effect on you. Your health and your appearance are like a wide-open book, every part of your body tells the story of your lives almost at first glance. I know when you look at people you can tell a million things about them too.

In the holistic world, it is said that your body shape is a direct reflection of whether you think positively or negatively about yourselves. The way you think of yourselves from the inside is what the outside world will accept you are. This is because you show it in your behaviour with your lack of confidence and bad opinion of yourselves.

You think millions of thoughts both good and bad, some kind and some completely unkind. They run through your minds every second through the day and night. These thoughts are powerful and sometimes brutal on your emotions, said with so much passion that they affect you physically and sometimes drain you of your energy.

Allowing these negative thoughts to run wildly and uncontrollably through your conscious mind, causes your subconscious mind, which believes anything the conscious mind tells it, to understand these thoughts as facts. Your conscious mind is a great ruminator, repeatedly making comments, like somebody sitting on your shoulder and constantly talking into your ear.

If for example as a rule you have a happy disposition and you smile and laugh a lot, your facial features reflect this. Frowning and being angry most of the time would reflect a completely different face. A happy face would have bright clear eyes with laughter lines around them, with your mouths curving up at the sides. As opposed to an angry face that shows scowl lines between your eyes, maybe even with the sides of your mouth dipping downwards and thin lips. The same applies to your body and health, being stressed and angry for long periods of time causes your body to release stress hormones like cortisol, oxidants and toxins into your blood stream, and over time this takes its toll on your physical health.

Having overdoses of these toxic substances released into your blood stream impacts the outcome of the development and rejuvenation of the cells in your bodies which renew themselves every two days. Oxidants cause havoc in your body. They are chemical reactions that transfer electrons or hydrogen from a substance to an oxidizing agent. Electrons and hydrogens are atoms that you are made up of. Every cell in your body is made up of these for energy transfer.

Oxidation reactions is a procedure that gives oxygen to other substances. This procedure damages and destroys cells and causes the release of free radicals. Free radicals are atoms that are made of nitrogen or oxygen with at least one damaged electron. In this case, you are talking about oxygen entered free radicals that were formed because of the splitting of weak molecule bonds. When they are free, they can start an undesirable chain reaction of connecting to other free radicals floating around in a cell causing it damage or death.

All the cells of your internal organs are only two days old or less, and you want to ensure that you stay healthy. To do this you need to supply your cells with the highest quality ingredients to renew themselves. This is good news, because this means you have the ability to have some control over your general health. Combining nutrition and exercise with positive thought control and stress reduction techniques, you assist your body to improve and get healthier as time goes by.

I know for some people reading this book it is hard to believe that simply by the thoughts you think, you affect your bodies. In quantum physics, you learn that your thoughts are vibrational energy right down to a molecular level. For your body to create energy to think or act, a molecular reaction has to occur for that energy to be activated. You think thoughts and feel emotions using your nervous system, which needs to produce energy to create your thoughts.

When someone you like walks into the room, your heart beats faster and your breathing quickens, the pupils of your eyes dilate, and you may even feel hot. You don't consciously control these reactions, but your bodies react before you are aware of it. This is all energy manufactured in your cells via the involuntary nervous system that is initiated by instructions from your central nervous system located in your brain.

As a personal fitness trainer, where the physical body is mainly focused on. Sometimes you forget that there is a whole wide world inside one physical body. Most of you don't relate to your inner self. Too often people who come to me for physical assistance, don't connect their physical problems with their emotional wellbeing. They are not aware that making changes to the way they think and to their lifestyle will jump start the physical changes they desire.

From my experience as a trainer I see that most of you are too busy and too distracted by your busy lives and hectic schedules. You find it hard to slow down and take the time to consider yourselves and ask why you look and feel the way you do. You are often impatient with yourselves. You get confused and don't understand why your bodies are not listening to you.

Why are you not perfect after all your gruelling workouts? Most of you are not aware that a punishing workout is not always going to get you results. Getting fit by compromising your body's health and putting it under so much stress is not recommended. If not replenished your body will get its eventual revenge and revert to its original weight and size.

The reality is that your bodies are trying to save your lives, this is its survival instinct that is built into your DNA. Investing in your health means taking the time to respectfully and lovingly, nurture yourselves with the right food, exercise and relaxation you need.

Chapter 3

Compensation and Body Image

Why do you over-train to boost your self-confidence?

Over the course of my career, I have seen many people working out. There are those who train for 4 or even 5 hours a day, every day for years. Over intense workouts are usually a very large indication of compensation for something going on in your lives that you are not happy about. This usually also indicates that you don't like the way you look and feel.

Over training is a disorder just like anorexia or bulimia. It could also be a result of a marital breakup, loss of a job, or any other stress situation that could beat up your confidence. Over training is a compensation to help you deal with issues that are difficult for you to handle.

Over trainers develop a strong and obsessional addiction to endorphins. If they are advised by medical experts for whatever reason to either stop working out or take a break from their workouts because of a sports injury, they would have powerful withdrawal symptoms, like anxiety, depression, restlessness, guilt, tension, loss of appetite, sleeplessness, and headaches.

Many exercisers develop an addiction to marathons, triathlons or iron man competitions. These are great events and a lot of fun when you are entering them for the right reasons, but too many people are obsessed with them. How can you tell the difference if you are obsessed or not? Usually you will see them working out without any rest periods, or they will insist on continuing their training suffering determinedly in spite of serious injuries. They will even continue to train excessively after they have been warned by a physician that continuing training in this condition could cause permanent damage.

It is easy to lose proportion of how long you should work out for, but the best indicator you have is your body. No pain no gain is out, if you have an injury or suffer from stress fractures or pain because of your workouts, you must listen to your body and stop. When somebody is addicted to their endorphin release, it is hard for them to slow down.

Their tendency to develop a desire to participate in every competition available despite their injuries is very common. They have a strong need to challenge themselves even more, above and beyond their limits. Overcoming their pain and injuries during their workout is equivalent to a personal trophy. There are limitations to the amount of competitions you should participate in, please live within these proportions.

Our bodies are not built for this amount of abuse. Even when training for the Olympics, athletes train with a very strict schedule designed specifically for competition seasons. They then go back to their regular workouts during non-competition seasons, preventing unnecessary injuries. People who over train keep training through all seasons, without a break for years. Harsh workouts while injured cause irreversible damage to their muscles, joints, ligaments, cartilage, skeleton and more. No matter how much pain they are in, they see it as a personal accomplishment when they get another workout in with their injury.

Food issues are also common. When I ask these clients about their diets, they answer way too quickly, telling me that they know how to eat well. This is an alarm bell. It worries me when they stress "really well," and I know it is not likely to be the case.

Some don't eat enough because they are afraid of messing up their currently achieved weight, they most likely lost weight through starvation and need to continue to starve to maintain this weight. Others feel because of their demanding workouts, they can eat "anything" and do, indulging in high calorie sugars and fats, so beginning their self-imposed yoyo maintenance challenge. Being disorganized, and not planning their meals ahead of time, is a classic recipe for disaster.

Planned meals allow for more efficient workouts, it also ensures that you are taking care of your body. Competitions like marathons, triathlons or iron man depletes your body of nutrients. This causes your body to go into what is called safe mode, this is where the body has now learned to store food as fat and from now on will no longer allow you to lose weight.

If your body works optimally, meaning that it is fed before it has to beg you to feed it, this is the most optimal situation. However, when you start to forget to eat, skip meals because you are busy, allowing your body to feel hunger pangs, this is your body begging for food. This starts a reaction that forces your body to activate its survival instinct and conserve energy. If you want to be athletes, then you should ensure that you worry about feeding and replenishing your bodies regularly.

Another type of over-trainer is where they eat very carefully, count every calorie, take supplements and also work out every day to the point of obsession. They get stressed and very anxious if they cannot train for any reason and tend to be inflexible. There are no compromises on their workout times, even at the expense of their family. Missing family events and even neglecting their responsibilities due to their workouts are common. This is a problem for a spouse or partner, because right now their life is all about them alone.

While they are in this excess training mode, this is the only focus in their lives. They will not go for drinks with friends, and restaurants are out of the question. Being a crucial member of a family, like a father or mother, who are not emotionally able to take responsibility for their share of family duties, builds resentments and will put a lot of stress on their relationship.

Some over-trainers are totally hooked on aerobics and do nothing else. They don't control their caloric intake believing there is no need for it because their aerobics forgives all food binges. They burst into the gym like a gale force wind and are always in a hurry, they are anxious to get started on their two-hour stint.

These people usually fixate on one specific treadmill, cross trainer or spinning bike that they love to workout with. They get upset or aggravated when the machine is being used by another gym member. They are not interested in logic and find it hard to divert to a different machine.

Over-trainers got results from their first few aerobic workouts, where they may have lost a respectable 20-30lbs, but now because of aerobic abuse, things have changed for them. It first started with slow weight gains and yoyoing to battle to not gain weight. After that their new battles with weight gain began, and there were always new baseline weights which they were striving to maintain. The final battle for them is usually after they have gained back all their weight and more, leaving them forever hopeful to get that huge loss they had once again.

Ultimately aerobic over-trainers show no long-term weight maintenance; however, they will never give up that original dream of their first glorious 20-30lbs weight loss. They have no understanding what is involved in achieving long-term weight loss and they succeeded in establishing their bodies into safe mode and are still waiting for miracles to happen.

Sometimes they do train with a workout program that incorporates muscle toning, aerobics and nutrition, but they always prefer to stick to their running. Too much aerobics is not healthy as there are too many risks for injuries, for example stress fractures, joint inflammation or joint damage due to abrasion of the repetitive motion you get from an aerobics workout.

Combined with poor nutrition and skipping meals, this is pure body abuse. Training like this are forces your body to go into safe mode and store all food as fat preventing you from losing weight. When you see exactly how to get thin, maybe you will be willing to give up some hours of your aerobics.

Aerobic workouts are only capable of "burning" calories during your workout, however if you are overdoing the aerobics this will not happen. This does cause frustration since now you are not seeing actual results from your arduous workout, so you resort to doing even more aerobics instead of less. Post workout, you should eat nutritiously rich foods, some believe that in the myth that calorie is a calorie, so it is not important what you eat, but the amount you eat. Meaning that if you eat a bar of chocolate with the same number of calories, proteins, carbohydrates and fat grams as a totally healthy and balanced meal, then what difference does it make, and the question is, does your body know the difference?

Of course, it does, because your body needs to find nutrients, vitamins and minerals from what you have eaten. If you chose to eat the chocolate bar, this is what your body is endeavouring to use to renew all the cells in your body. This is why it is said you are what you eat.

THE ART OF POSITIVE THINKING AND BODY IMAGE

Cells in your bodies spark your desires and thoughts in a two-way communication system from your brain toy our cells and from your cells back to your brain. This communication transpires via your central nervous system, where you have voluntary and involuntary nerves located in your spinal cord. By using vibrational energy, your brain transmits instructional thoughts through your nervous system. This is the simple reason why you don't have to tell your lungs to breathe and your heart to beat, it is controlled by the involuntary nervous system.

Your brain transmits information down the spinal cord, which the nerve cells transfer to your muscles, organs and all over your body including fat cells. Fat cells also transmit information. They transmit the desire to get filled because they are responsible for your survival. If you have not been eating regularly, the fat cells communicate to your brain that you are hungry, your brain makes you crave fattening sugary foods and you eat without control to refill the fat cells.

When you are a normal weight, under normal circumstances your fat cells secrete a hormone called leptin which triggers receptors on hypothalamic nerve cells, which leads to decreased hunger and you don't go on a food search. Leptin is a hormone in charge of your appetite and generally regulates your body fat via your hunger sensations.

Your body is an amazing machine, all your systems work precisely and intrinsically all communicating and coordinating with perfect synchronization so that you stay alive. How does your arm move? By your brain thinking first, your brain sends a message down the spinal cord, through the voluntary nerves to your arm and it moves, via thoughts through your nervous system. This whole process takes a fraction of a second.

You are not even aware you decided to move your arm before you moved it. All these things happen in your body without you having to consciously worry about the logistics. You also have fine motor functions, like when you want to use your fingers intricately to play a musical instrument for example, you don't have to think how to move your fingers over the piano keys. Your brain coordinates and instructs the motor neurons which muscles to ignite, and in what sequence.

You are responsible for your thoughts so that you think positive and send positive messages into your body. You can literally think yourselves sick or you can choose to think yourselves healthy. Your body needs all the help it can get to help it maintain healthy levels of hormones, chemicals and pH balance.

Love yourself and respect yourself, admire your achievements and invest in your emotional and physical health. I know you want to get rid of that sedentary look, and it is so possible if you do it right, and the secret is getting it right.

Use this book to guide you toward choosing the right nutrition by learning about food that suits you and combining it with the appropriate amount of aerobics and muscle training. You will also address stress and gastrointestinal related problems and learn about foods that will reduce symptoms and help heal problems giving your body a chance to reset. But the hard work must come from you.

Chapter 4

Stress Mode

To lose weight you must understand why you are not.
Stress is the most likely root cause of what is keeping you fat. The world is stressful, and this extreme stress awakens biological changes and reactions in your body. A brutally fast paced lifestyle combined with all the responsibilities and commitments take their toll on your bodies. You work too many hours and don't get enough rest or sleep.

When was the last time you stopped to give yourself a break, maybe a massage, or even a day at the spa? You usually can't afford to take time off from work, the simple fact is that if you don't work you don't get paid. Your lifestyles come with huge bills and taxes usually from necessities and not even luxuries. The result is as the years go by your workload and responsibilities get bigger and your free time gets scarcer.

THERE ARE TWO STAGES TO YOUR REACTIONS TO STRESS

The first stage is what you call the catabolic reaction, which causes wild biological changes to your body. This stress reaction causes your system to not be able to use food as an energy source, forcing your body live off itself, which makes you lose weight at first. With the catabolic reaction, you have lost your appetite and you are constantly burning energy because your body is so completely stressed.

Our body cannot keep up with the amount calories necessary for it to get through this period. Your intestines are affected by your lack of interest in food. What is happening in your body is a much faster heart rate, your body is in a constant state of tension, alarm and alertness. Your breathing is much faster, and your body has a much higher demand for oxygen, it is like you are doing aerobics 24 hours a day. You also feel hot and sweaty and the combination of all these symptoms is that you burn so many calories. In this stage of stress your body breaks down fibres at a very fast pace.

You lose a lot of weight with this reaction and you may get skinny because your bodies are producing adrenaline, which is also known as the panic hormone, at such a fast pace. The panic hormone is released into your bodies in huge quantities as though you have undergone a huge trauma, like a car accident. This disrupts your metabolism and disrupts your body's production of protein, fats and carbohydrates.

Because your body increases the production of fast energy this causes your body to lose the proteins, potassium, phosphorus and magnesium from the muscle fibres and you lose a lot of weight, which also means your body stores less calcium in your bones, risking osteoporosis. In this situation, your body absorbs fewer nutritional components from your diet, especially Vitamin B which has an important role in protecting the nervous system.

After a certain amount of time of being in first the stage stress reaction, your body's strong survival instinct stops this avalanche, and takes you into the second stage of your biological reaction to stress.

The second stage that occurs in your body's reaction to stress is called the cortisol or insulin reaction. In this reaction stage your body will try to repair all the damage done by the catabolic reaction. This means that huge amounts of insulin are released into your body causing you now to gain weight. Your body will start to try and protect itself by opposing the tension and stress.

It will try to stabilize itself by stopping the breakdown procedure by encouraging the release of anabolic hormones, which is insulin. With the high level of cortisol in your system the adrenaline level is forced to lower. The insulin, which is basically steroids, tries to combat the catabolic procedure by desperately trying to gain weight.

How does it do this? By lowering your heart rate significantly to a more efficient pace in order for your body to conserve energy. Now you are burning too few calories and your body starts "winning" the battle for survival and you are gaining weight back and fast. Being in survival mode is what is known as fight or flight, which is a neuronal and hormonal stress response from your nervous system.

Our blood pressure also lowers, and your breathing is much slower as opposed to the catabolic reaction. Your body now requires less oxygen, you have very low energy and you now don't sweat. This reaction stage to stress takes much longer to pass than the catabolic stage. The new insulin level in your system ensures that you stay heavier, which is also the reason why you may be steadily gaining weight.

For some of you this stage could last years. I know people that are in this stage and I know this is a catch 22 situation, when you are heavy you don't want to eat, but if you don't eat your body will gain even more weight. When your body is in survival mode, this means your body is out of sync and desperately trying to save your lives. Remember balance is so important, your store balance by making sure to eat every 3 hours or so.

As a rule, whenever your body is off balance and out of sync you pay a high price with your health. So, it is important to take care of yourselves and make sure you don't get into these extreme reactions.

HOW DO YOU GET SO STRESSED?

Physical causes like sickness, operations or accidents.

Environmental causes like poisoning from microorganisms, exposure to heat or cold, pollution, radiation and strong noises.

Mental causes like stress at work, financial stress, sickness, death of a family member or close friend.

You lose control of your time and personal space by allowing other people like your bosses, spouses, children and friends to have too much control over your lives and dictate how you utilize your time. You think that you will take a vacation next year, and you just keep on pushing your bodies until...when?

Because of these stresses that comes with a hectic lifestyle, your body feels the enormous pressure and must protect itself. It then goes through the two stages of stress reactions you now know are first stage by closing all metabolism and releasing adrenaline, second stage by releasing huge amounts of insulin into your body. This chemical imbalance between your adrenaline and insulin levels causes havoc to all your bodily systems.

There is no harmony or synchronization within or between each of your systems. The blood stream which distributes nutrients, has no nutrients to circulate. The digestive tract can't metabolize food, the liver can't secrete bile or filter toxins and the pancreas is overloaded with cortisol.

When your body feels, it is not being taken care of it takes this as a threat to its survival. It has no choice but to go into stress mode, which you now know is your survival system. It is like the airbag in your car being released while you are still driving. Stress displays itself as disease.

Issues like body weight, high blood pressure, heart problems, free radicals and oxidants floating in your blood stream, will cause a stress reaction from your body, any of which may develop into more serious unwanted diseases and more. You have many organs that are susceptible to extreme stress and can fail. Usually the first to suffer and the primary cause of disease is in your digestive tract, the stomach, the bowel, and the small and large intestines. They have a problem working under pressure and start having blockages that damage their wall linings.

As a result, you are not liking the way you look and feel, and because you feel so bad about yourselves you start thinking negatively, and your body image goes further downhill and you start to think unhealthy and unproductive thoughts. This is a chain reaction your unhealthy thinking causes high levels of stress which may open the door for diseases to develop.

These negative thoughts could also affect negatively the outcome of the sensitive cell division procedure, which then may cause free radicals to be released and oxidation of electrons or hydrogens. Your body craves sugars to keep up its level of cortisol which it needs to maintain your stress reaction. Levels of insulin rise even more because of this craving for sugar without control, and your weight keeps creeping up. So, exercise and diet are the answer but not completely, this situation needs to be treated differently.

Under normal situations when a person is overweight because of overeating, the logical calculation per all the fitness experts, is if you eat less than you burn then you should lose weight. But to be fair, most people who are overweight suffer from abnormal emotional stresses. An overweight body is an obvious symptom to a cause which needs to be discovered.

The harsh calculation of eating less than you burn in these cases is not relevant and it is not fair. Your physical and your emotional wellbeing are connected in every situation. If someone is overweight or has bad skin or anything else, treating only the symptom is not going to cure the source of the problem. If the source of the problem is not discovered or treated, then the symptom becomes a recurring issue. The only way to discover the source of the problem and solve it is by considering the complete picture, and relating to the whole person, this allows you to discover the root of the problem.

It is very possible to achieve your goal weight and health. The first stage is the decision to take control of yourselves by committing to the long process leading to complete health. Understanding that eating healthy food, taking time to relax and working out, is very individual, and so is everyone's progress level.

You don't need to take an expensive vacation to Hawaii to relax. You can learn to relax utilizing even little pockets of free time you have with a positive attitude and mind-set. You may discover you can relax even while working, finding out that vacation is really a mind-set using relaxation techniques. Everyone does what they can, and it is all okay. Some people will take baby steps and others will do a complete change over immediately.

Chapter 5

Safe Mode

Safe mode really means survival mode.

Understanding your body is an art that you are not necessarily born with, for some of you it may take a lifetime and for others not. Becoming attuned to your body is the important thing. Taking care of it is a balancing act which you learn over time. Since your body also constantly changes as a reaction to life situations, keeping up with it may be difficult. Taking time to listen to your bodily needs by feeding and nourishing your body is critical.

It is also best to keep away from huge meals or junk food. The ideal method is small meals at regular intervals. This is a great way to start a healing process. The result of years of imbalance causes your metabolism to malfunction. Your body then becomes a master at storing food into your fat cells. Understanding your body and how it functions gives you a better picture of how you ended up looking the way you do. This is the only body you have to take you through your lives.

Not taking care of it then this forces your body to protect itself, and when it does, you don't like the results. Your body protects you by not allowing you to "waste" calories at all, it views any weight loss as a serious malfunction and must protect you immediately. It does this by using the only survival technique it knows, which is conserving and rationing your fat supply. This protection system is called "safe mode," which means that your body is very frugal with how it allows you to use its carefully stored fat.

Once your body is forced to protect itself, the procedure of getting yourself out of safe mode could be very long and drawn out. This needs a lot of patience and determination. I understand that it is frustrating if you don't always see results as quickly as you want. But healing yourself from safe mode is a reverse process. Your body is recovering from a serious situation that took you a long time to get to.

Also, in safe mode, you feel that your body is out of your control, which it really is. Your body is trying to gain back control internally. All your systems are completely out of sync as a result of bad eating habits. So, when you continue to eat irregularly and go for many hours without food or nourishment, you are not allowing your body to recover and regain order over its territories. Another consequence of not eating for many hours is the complete loss of control over your body's hunger and demand immediate satiation.

So, you eat everything in sight and more. This is totally confusing for your body and a recipe for disaster, your body craves regularity and consistency. The longer your body stays in survival mode, the worse your body composition gets. This just makes the situation much worse. This is the dieting cycle you get into, and with each revolution of the cycle you lose more muscle and essential proteins and gain more fat.

HOW MANY TIMES HAVE YOU STARVED YOURSELF IN ORDER TO LOSE WEIGHT?

I bet more times than you can remember. I also know that you are aware of how detrimental and harmful this is for your body. Each time you starve your body it is forced to feed itself from your own body. This is called catabolism, using your muscles or other crucial proteins, connective tissues and collagen as food sources. One example is, elastin which are connective tissues found in and around your internal organs, holding them in place.

Starving behaviour also forces your body to store food as fat. Your body understands regularity, when food does not arrive as expected your body will store any food you eat as fat. Only until it learns to trust us, which is approximately a few months after you have started eating regularly, will your body start to allow you to lose fat.

Fat is the most durable material in your body, designed to survive difficult times like famine. Fat cells influence your appetite via the nervous system and a hormone called leptin. The fact is fat cells are designed to grow. Each fat cell always desires to be fatter because that is the way it is programmed in your DNA for survival. They do this by causing you to desire to eat chocolate or something rich in fat and sugar in order to get fatter. Therefore, sometimes you cannot control or resist what you are eating.

Losing weight through starvation, or irregular eating habits very much stresses out your fat cells. They start sending out alarms signals to all your bodily systems informing them that there is a shortage of food. Your body reacts promptly and efficiently by slowing down all your bodily functions and systems. Your BMR, basal metabolic rate is now set at a very reduced pace to conserve energy and calories.

This is the number of calories your body needs daily for life support, which is now drastically reduced. This forces your body to find calories from within itself, which it takes from your crucial proteins. Proteins are much harder for you to gain, so losing them is really a huge loss. Your fat cells have a powerful influence over your nervous system, causing strong cravings for fattening foods immediately. When this desire is sent to your brains, believe me you have no control over what you eat.

It is a vicious cycle. You have a bad body image because you are not in optimal condition. This causes an interruption of your natural metabolism, because of irregular behaviour with food and lifestyle and the desire to lose weight fast. Thus, your body goes into the safe mode reaction process, which is the opposite of your desired intention.

The result being, you become overweight with bad skin, thinning hair and general bad health. When you don't eat as you should, you don't have enough healthy nutrients and calories in your body for you to function optimally. At the same time, you are also overfed because you eat too much non-nutritious junk foods. You eat fast food or junk food instead of healthy food because your fat cells are demanding food, fast and in large quantities. The result is that your body starts to look the way you don't like.

HOW DO YOU LOSE WEIGHT?

Losing weight is not easy once your body is in safe mode, I really do know and understand that. After training many people over the years, I can say it is really patience and consistency that awards you the ultimate results. The most important and helpful thing to remember is that your body is an amazing and logically functioning miracle. You owe your body so much respect and awe, to understand why it behaves the way it does. Give it the benefit of the doubt, because ultimately all your body is trying to do is keep you alive and safe.

If you understand that your body is a rhythmic being and all of your bodily systems work in cycles, you would really appreciate why your body craves routine, rhythm and stability. Every system works within itself in a cycle, like the heart, blood, lungs etc. Between themselves is also another very intricate and complicated cycle, combining coordination, synchronization and timing, which your body does with amazing precision and proficiency. If you oversaw organizing your systems consciously, you would have messed it up a long time ago.

The lungs cleanse, warm and soften the oxygen you breathe, and are also in charge of oxygenation of blood.

The heart pumps blood full of Co2 (Carbon Dioxide) from the body into the lungs, and from the lungs filled with oxygen into your body.

The blood stream, rich in oxygen from the heart and nutrients from your digestive tract, distributes nourishment and oxygen to all your organs.

The digestive system breaks down and sorts out all of the food you eat, deciding what to use and what to store and what to send out to waste.

Our liver oversees detoxifying and filtering out all the toxins from your blood stream by producing bile.

The pancreas produces and balances hormones such as your insulin level. It also secretes pancreatic juice containing digestive enzymes that assist digestion and absorption of nutrients in the small intestine.

The skin is the largest organ of your body and has multiple layers of ectodermal tissue that protects your muscles, bones, ligaments and internal organs. It is also in charge of sensation, heat regulation, evaporation, excretion, and water resistance.

Every one of your organs are made up of millions of cells that renew themselves every two days.

The nervous system starts with the brain, which oversees making sure the body is functioning via involuntary nerves. You use the voluntary nerves and motor neurons for conscious actions, like walking, eating, etc. your body is also always in sync with nature.

You inhale oxygen and exhale carbon dioxide, and the plants and trees inhale carbon dioxide and exhale oxygen for us.

The earth rotates around the sun and the moon orbits the earth. The earth is always spinning and tilted at exactly 23.4° while remaining completely in sync with the sun and moon. All three circle at the perfect pace, taking the perfect amount of time that is needed to ensure that the sun and moon maintain life on earth.

If this perfect harmony was disturbed and the moon, for example, started circling the earth faster or slower, this would upset the earth's atmosphere and earth would no longer be rich in oxygen, vitamins and minerals that enable organisms to live.

When you upset your body tempo you confuse and disorientate your body. Taken off balance, there is an avalanche effect on all your systems, since each system relies on the next, they all start crashing down. Losing control, your body starts to send out panicked alert signals in the desperate effort to save your life, sending your body into safe mode.

Even though your body is a miracle, the process of losing weight is not a miracle as such. Those of you who have been battling weight problems for years already know this. It takes total dedication and commitment. But once you decide and commit to go all the way, the results are even better than you ever dreamed of.

THERE ARE 3 CRUCIAL ELEMENTS TO THE WEIGHT LOSS PROCESS SYSTEM:

⇒ Nutrition
⇒ Muscle mass
⇒ Aerobics

Now I stressed crucial because just doing 2 out of the 3 elements will not work. And if it seems like it is working at first, it really isn't. Weight loss you would be experiencing in this way, is the same weight loss type that happens during the first stage of the stress reaction.

This "weight loss" will be very difficult to maintain, since your body then triggers its fight or flight survival mode and goes into the second stage of stress. Remember fight or flight is a cortisol reaction that prevents weight loss by drastically increasing its levels making you gain weight.

This is the trigger of a vicious cycle which you don't want. Some people may spend a lifetime going from safe mode into stress mode and back again. Sadly, this is the reason why you always seem to have to battle with your weight. the way to ensure you get the results you desire is making sure you do it right, which means not to starve yourselves and eating even though it does feel like that is defeating the purpose.

Maintenance, rhythm and routine are what your bodies crave, because all of your bodily systems work in cycles. When your body is permitted to work as it should, staying the same weight for years is possible and the dedication and effort is so worth it.

NUTRITION

Nutrition is probably the most important element of this triangle. Most of you don't take nutrition seriously enough, and to be honest as long as you don't have any adverse reactions to any food types, and you are healthy there is no reason why you should. You don't have diabetes, and you also don't suffer from gastrointestinal diseases, so it is easy to be lazy and continue as you are used to. Eating healthy is always something you promise you will do in the future, and hopefully before you get sick. But you are what you eat even if you do seem to be healthy.

In fact, you really do believe that you are eating well enough, but if you are honest with yourselves, you must admit it is very difficult to spot your own mistakes and understand why you will not lose weight if you continue to eat as you have been. Your nutritional needs are so specific and should be adjusted per your own unique body. For those of you who own cars, if for example, you have a Mazda 3 with a 1.6 engine that needs a certain oil you won't buy an oil suitable for a Nissan Micra with a 1.2 engine.

Understanding every individual is unique, a nutrition program your best friend got from her nutritionist is not good for you. I know it is more economical and convenient to just photocopy your friend's nutrition plan, but her chemistry is different from yours. Her nutrition plan is a chemical reaction to her personal chemistry. Your blood test results will most certainly be different from hers. Your blood tests will indicate what you need.

MUSCLE MASS

Muscle mass is another element that is essential for permanent weight loss. the more muscle you have, the easier you will lose weight and stay lean. Muscle mass is what you lose a lot of when your body is in safe mode, since it is the main energy source your body has been using to survive.

It is crucial to try and build up and recover your muscle mass and say "thank you" to any muscle mass you can gain. This is what will protect you over the next coming years.

Women are afraid of getting too muscular and know that an exercise program in the gym is designed to build muscle mass. But muscle mass is a crucial factor for maintaining an ideal body weight and raising your BMR.

Working in gyms for over 20 years, I saw how long it takes for guys to build muscle mass. They work hard for their muscles, not to mention all the protein shakes, gainers and chemicals they may take to achieve their goal. It takes most guys with decent genetics approximately two years of intense and dedicated workouts to get bulked.

Women don't bulk up that easily, but the fact is, having more muscle mass changes your body composition so that you burn more calories per hour. This is the simple reason why guys lose weight in seconds and women just look at food and gain weight. The fact is that the more muscle mass you have the leaner you will be.

"A KITTEN WILL NEVER GROW INTO A LION" NO MATTER HOW HARD IT WORKS OUT.

Everyone has a natural built-in peak level which when reached, your muscles will cease to enlarge. This is the miracle of nature, to ensure that you don't just grow and grow thanks to a protein called myostatin. The less you have of this protein the more muscular you get. You all have your own personal levels of testosterone and myostatin. Combined with genetics, this determines how big you get.

When you reach your maximum amount of muscle mass, and you want to really bulk up more, you need to take protein shakes, Creatine and other supplements.

Steroids also raises testosterone levels, but please don't touch this stuff, it really messes up your system, and can cause problems like high cholesterol, acne, and high blood pressure. Steroids also thickens the left ventricle wall of your heart, meaning you will have a higher risk of heart attacks and strokes.

It is also hard on your liver and kidneys, and you risk severe liver damage. Steroids from un-natural sources forces your body to have to deal with all the foreign chemicals very large doses. It's a shame for a healthy person interested in their health and aesthetics to damage themselves for no great reason.

AEROBICS

Aerobics is the part of the triple action that you must be the most careful with. There are a lot of myths surrounding

41

aerobic exercise, too many people think that this is the main element that causes you to lose weight. I wish I could sign you all to a legal contract that does not allow you to work out for longer than 60 minutes' aerobics. Too much aerobics has adverse results which I know surprises you, but it has it's benefits in the right amounts. I know you are asking "but doesn't aerobics burn the calories?" – well, not necessarily.

When you go on the elliptical machine for 3 hours and it reads that you burned 3,000 calories, it is simply not true. Here's why. If, for example, the machine tells you that you burned 600 calories in the first hour, the second hour will be less and the third hour even less – that is a physiological fact.

Our body is a great energy conserver and a survivor, so as you are working out your body mechanics are getting more efficient at whatever motion you are doing. It does this by not wasting energy on extra movements. For example, with every revolution of the elliptical trainer your body learns to perform more effortlessly and over time, getting to know the machine and your biomechanics during the workout well enough to anticipate the motions.

You conserve energy as you get adjusted to a machine or other forms of aerobics, so each time you work out your body burns less calories than the last time. The computer on the elliptical machine or treadmill is only a computer, it makes a logical calculation, but it is not measuring an actual human body. It is really calculating the number of watts the machine is using. Another fact is that your body saves energy and calories when it sees a lot of calories being used, it takes it as a warning that something is wrong in the body and may go into safe mode.

The sad fact is that a fat body does not burn fat it stores it. Not willing to depart from its fat stores until you stabilize your body combining nutrition, muscle mass and aerobics. If you are overweight and have stayed overweight even though you work out for hours on aerobics machines every day for years. You must ask yourself "why are you not losing weight?" Good question. You have now come to the realization that your body is not burning calories at all because it is in safe mode.

Chapter 6

What IS Fat?

Let's look at this material we call fat.

You are so focused on how unattractive fat makes you feel and look, you then forget why your body composition includes fat. Why do you need fat? You ask, fat cells known as adipose tissue is made from cells called adipocytes.

Fat is an excellent protector and insulator, it cushions your body under your skin and keeps your internal organs in place and prevents drastic heat loss this is what is known as essential body fat, which is necessary to maintain your life and reproductive functions.

You store fat under your skin (called subcutaneous fat) and in your body cavity around your internal organs (called visceral fat). Fat together with your liver stores Vitamin D in your subcutaneous fat and releases it into your blood stream slowly as you need it. Your brain and nerve cells rely on fat and in fact your prime source of energy is from glucose which your body uses to produce fat. Triglycerides are stored in your fat cells, when they expand in diameter and get larger, they make you look fat. Triglycerides are important for energy reserves, these fat cells secrete chemicals that play a part in your appetite, protects nerve tissue, and help regulate women's menstrual cycles.

The pancreas releases enzymes called lipases that attack the surface of each fat molecule and break the fats down into two parts, glycerol and fatty acids. Because fat molecules are too big to easily cross cell membranes, the fat cells must be broken down first. This ensures that they pass from the intestine through the intestinal cells into the lymphatic system, or any cell barrier.

These fat cells are called lipoprotein, they transport dietary lipids (fats) from the intestines to various areas in your body. They also enable fats and cholesterol to be transported in your water-based bloodstream. Lipoprotein lipase break the fats into fatty acids and are found in the blood vessels walls. The fatty acids are then absorbed from the blood into fat cells, muscle cells and liver cells. Once in the liver, the glycerol and fatty acids can be either further broken down or used to make glucose.

THE DIFFERENCES THE WAY MEN AND WOMEN STORE FAT

The hormone Oestrogen causes fat to be stored around the pelvis (hips), the buttocks and thighs in women, men on the other hand tend to store visceral fat around their bellies. This sex-specific fat, as it is known for women, is supposed to be a physiological advantage during pregnancies. Women's bodies are more efficient at storing fat because their bodies are always in preparation for fertility, foetal development and lactation.

This is known as the healthy fat, even though it is not aesthetic, it is because women have larger fat cells around the gluteal, pelvic and thigh area which you know as cellulite.

The rate of body fat accumulation particularly sex-specific fat is attributed mostly to changes in female hormone levels, such as prolactin and oxytocin required for lactation (nursing). Sex-specific fat cells around the hips and thighs increase their fat-releasing activity and decrease their storage capacity. While at the same time fat storage increases in the mammary adipose tissue.

So basically, the fat stores from the hips and thighs are now being used to produce milk, women tend to deposit fat in their bodies during pregnancy and lose it during lactation.

Men tend to store excess fat in the visceral, or abdominal area. Not only is this not an advantage, it is dangerous and even life threatening. A large belly, where the waist circumference is larger than the hip girth, is strongly associated with an increased risk of coronary artery disease, diabetes, elevated triglycerides, hypertension, cancer and risk of early mortality.

Women have a lower basal fat oxidation rate because their body composition is made up of less muscle mass, their BMR is much lower than men. Men actually lose weight easier than women because of their high muscle mass ratio to fat, even when they are resting men burn more calories than women.

The reason is hormonal, men have testosterone which causes them to have more muscle mass and less percentage of body fat. Women have oestrogen which causes them to store more fat which they need physiologically. Women store 11% more body fat than men, even women body builders never get to below 6% body fat.

Women must do a lot more exercise if they would like to achieve the same health benefits as men, this includes both diet and exercise. Even though exercise alone might be enough for men to lose weight, women need to take their caloric intake into consideration also.

LOSING WEIGHT FROM LOSING FAT

As you know too much fat besides being unattractive, is not healthy and causes a lot of problems. Being too fat causes clogged arteries, heart disease and high risk for heart attacks and diabetes. It is so important for you to regulate your cortisol levels by controlling your behaviour pattern towards food and get into a healthy lifestyle as part of your daily routine.

Our weight is determined by the rate which you store energy from the food that you eat, and the rate at which you use that energy. Your body breaks down fat as you lose weight, but you cannot reduce the number of fat cells you have. You will always have the same number or fat cells you were born with. As you lose weight each fat cell simply gets smaller and as you gain weight your fat cells expand.

Fat cells are your body's emergency storage, they store fuel for you just in case you need it later on to survive. If you didn't have fat cells, you wouldn't have survived the famines of the past. During the Holocaust, the people who survived were the ones who had a larger fat store. Fat cells are a sophisticated survival mechanism that is unfortunately getting all the wrong signals today. Your body was not designed for the constant intake of food, especially the processed junk food that contains preservatives and high levels of sugar.

Maintaining a stable weight currently takes a lot more effort compared to your parents' generation. You live in a world with too much abundance of junk food, stress, financial responsibilities and sedentariness. You are however exposed to an abundance of information and awareness of what a healthy lifestyle is supposed to be. You are more educated than your parents about exercise and nutrition, you do know that you should be doing physical activity every day and try to eat healthy.

Chapter 7

Medications

Antidepressants and other medications

Medications scare me and relying on medications terrifies me. I know that doctors make a lot of money in commission when administering drugs. If you have to take medications please check and double check that you really need them, or you may have a problem getting off of them later on.

Antidepressants are very addictive; you cannot just come off of them cold turkey. It is a long and drawn out procedure. While taking antidepressants, people are not always aware that they are addicted to them, much like a smoker if asked he will tell you he can stop smoking tomorrow if he wants to. Only when he tries to stop does he realize that he can't, the same goes for antidepressants.

Medications are chemicals that react with your chemistry, they are in your blood stream and infiltrate every cell in your body becoming part of your DNA. Therefore, they can change your personality, change your body shape and your emotional reactions to life.

Most medications taken are not necessary. A lot of times doctors give you drugs because it is easier to medicate than to check out what the real problem is. Doctors don't connect mind and body, they just treat the body, and then only one small part of it. The trouble is that they don't really

49

care about your welfare, even though they believe they do. They don't see your life down the road and say, "this poor person must deal with weaning themselves off these drugs one day."

Doctors know and understand the poison that is in these medications, and they know the damage these powerful drugs due to your liver. Their calculation is between the affects your depression has on your emotional state and your coping skills with life now.

People suffering from bi-polar or schizophrenia or any other psychotic illnesses, do need their medications. Just like epileptic persons must take their medications carefully. If you suffer from any disorder or disease that you need to take medication to live normally, always take your medications on time as your physician ordered.

There are situations where you feel slightly blue and you go to your doctor for help, after which he decides that you need antidepressants. Be careful, and know that there are natural alternatives, such as herbs, Bach flower remedies and aromatherapy. Taking natural products that help you cope with temporary situations like these that are not addicting. Most times stressing situations are not permanent, and you don't need to be taking treatments forever.

You all need help occasionally and that is okay, and if you do then it is always better to go the natural route in these situations. Living a natural life medication free is the optimal, using healing herbs from natural sources only when you need them. It is always best to allow your body to function normally and not to encourage it to rely on help for long periods of time.

Even multivitamins are only taken as a reinforcement and backup in case you are not able to get all the nutrients you need from nutrition only. Taking supplements are great if you are going through a hard time, or you have been sick, and your body needs some assistance. It is always better to get your vitamins from food sources first. When you eat a healthy and balanced diet it is possible.

People suffering from liver diseases, asthma, severe joint inflammation diseases or any other similar conditions that steroids are administered for, are taking steroid medications. These are usually corticosteroids, and they have many undesirable and dangerous side effects, one being weight gain. These sufferers may get bloated looking like they were blown up like a balloon.

It is very difficult to get thin while taking these medications, so if you need to take this medication, try and stay on an anti-stress nutrition lifestyle to reduce the amount of weight you gain. When you come off the medication it will not be so hard to get back on track.

Maintaining balanced nutrition, light exercise daily and relaxing as much as you can. This does not mean in front of the television all day long. Go to classes such as yoga, Feldenkrais, Pilates, stretch, water aerobics or any other form of activity that I have listed in this book designed to lower your heart rate and reduce your stress levels.

The goal is to get yourself healthy and try and get off chemical medications. And don't give up ever!

Chapter 8

Diabetes, what exactly is it

DIABETES IS A CHRONIC LONG-TERM CONDITION

This is a condition marked by abnormally high levels of sugar glucose in the blood. People with diabetes either do not produce enough insulin, which is a hormone needed to convert sugar, starches and other foods into energy needed for daily life or cannot use the insulin that their bodies produce. As a result, the glucose builds up in the bloodstream and if it is left untreated, the diabetes can lead to blindness, kidney disease, nerve disease, heart disease, and stroke.

According to the National Institute of Diabetes and Digestive and Kidney Diseases (NIDDK), diabetes affects 25.8 million Americans. While an estimated 18.8 million have been diagnosed with diabetes of both types, 1 and type 2, unfortunately, nearly one third of people are unaware that they have type 2 diabetes. Diabetes is widely recognized as one of the leading causes of death and disability.

A Pre-diabetes conditions occurs in individuals with blood glucose levels that are higher than normal but not high enough for a diagnosis of diabetes. This condition raises the risk of developing type 2 diabetes, stroke, and heart disease. In fact, people with diabetes are sometimes more likely than non-diabetic people to develop heart disease.

Pre-diabetes is also called impaired fasting glucose (IFG), impaired glucose tolerance (IGT), or insulin resistance. Some people have both IFG and IGT. In IFG, glucose levels are a little high several hours after a person eats. In IGT, glucose levels are a little higher than normal right after eating. Pre-diabetes is becoming more common Many individuals who suffer with pre-diabetes are likely to go on to develop type 2 diabetes within ten years. Diabetes may also be associated with genetic syndromes, surgery, drugs, malnutrition, infections, and other illnesses.

THERE ARE 2 MAJOR TYPES OF DIABETES

Type 1 diabetes - Also known as juvenile or insulin dependent diabetes, this type of diabetes occurs when the cells of the pancreas that are responsible for producing insulin are destroyed by the immune system. As a result, the pancreas permanently loses its ability to produce enough insulin to regulate blood sugar levels appropriately. Type 1 diabetes is usually diagnosed in early childhood and can be managed but cannot be cured.

SIGNS AND SYMPTOMS
Type 1 diabetes can occur at any age, but it usually starts in people younger than thirty. These symptoms are usually severe and occur rapidly.

⇒ Increased thirst
⇒ Increased urination
⇒ Weight loss despite increased appetite
⇒ Nausea
⇒ Vomiting
⇒ Abdominal pain

⇒ Fatigue

⇒ Absence of menstruation

FAMILY HISTORY OF TYPE 1 DIABETES

A mother who had pre-eclampsia, a condition that happens in pregnancy that has a sharp increase in blood pressure during the third trimester of pregnancy. There is usually family history of autoimmune diseases, including Hashimoto's thyroiditis, Graves' disease, myasthenia gravis, Addison's disease, or pernicious anaemia. If there were viral infections during infancy, including mumps, rubella, and coxsackie, a child of an older mother, of Northern European or Mediterranean descent, or even a lack of being breastfed.

CAUSES

Both type 1 and type 2 diabetes are caused by the absence, insufficient production, or lack of response by cells in the body to the hormone insulin. Insulin is a key regulator of the body's metabolism. After meals, food is digested in the stomach and intestines. Sugar which are glucose molecules, are absorbed directly into the bloodstream and blood glucose levels rise. Under normal circumstances, the rise in blood glucose levels signals specific cells in the pancreas called beta cells, they secrete insulin into the bloodstream. Insulin then enables the glucose to enter the cells in the body that may be burned for energy or stored for future use.

In type 1 diabetes, the beta cells of the pancreas produce little or no insulin of the hormone that allows glucose to enter body cells. Once glucose enters a cell, it is used as fuel. When there is not adequate insulin, the glucose builds up in the bloodstream instead of going into the cells. The body is unable to use this glucose for energy despite the high levels in the bloodstream, this leads us to experience increased hunger. In addition, the high levels of glucose in the blood causes us to urinate more, which then leads to excessive thirst. After much time like this the insulin-producing beta cells of the pancreas can become destroyed and unable to produce insulin.

The truth is that exact cause of type 1 diabetes is not known, and each year more and more young people are being diagnosed with type 1 diabetes.

Unfortunately, there is no proven way to prevent type 1 diabetes. However, some research in Finland suggests that providing adequate amounts of vitamin D in the first years of your child's life, may decrease their chances of developing type 1 diabetes. In northern Finland where there is almost no sunlight, researchers followed 10,000 infants for thirty years, those given at least 2,000 IU of vitamin D per day for the first year of their life were significantly less likely to develop type 1 diabetes than infants who were given less than that. Other studies have confirmed that doses of 2,000 IU or higher of vitamin D may have a strong protective effect against type 1 diabetes.

Type 2 diabetes – This form of the disease makes up 90% or more of all cases of diabetes and usually develops in adulthood. It occurs when the pancreas cannot make enough insulin to keep blood glucose levels normal. Unfortunately, it is made worse by poor food choices, a sedentary lifestyle, and being overweight. Diabetes is a serious condition, and sadly many people with type 2 diabetes do not know they have it. It is becoming more common due to the increase in obesity and failure to exercise. The brutal truth is that Type 2 diabetes can be improved and even reversed by the simple decision and commitment to lifestyle changes. Adopting a healthy diet, becoming more active, and losing excess weight.

This form of diabetes usually develops in older, overweight individuals who become resistant to the effects of insulin over time. When it is diagnosed, the pancreas is usually producing enough insulin but, for unknown reasons, the body cannot use the insulin effectively. This is called insulin resistance and means that the insulin produced by your pancreas cannot connect with fat and muscle cells to let glucose inside and produce energy, this causes hyperglycaemia, which is a high blood glucose. So to compensate, the pancreas feels it needs to produces even more insulin. The cells sense this flood of insulin and become even more resistant, resulting in a vicious cycle of high glucose levels and often high insulin levels.

Inflammation is also common among people with type 2 diabetes. Inflammatory markers are chemicals in the body that lead to inflammation, such as interleukin-6 and C-reactive proteins, have been found to be increased in those with type 2 diabetes. This diabetes usually creeps up on us gradually, even though it mainly happens to overweight people, it can also develop in lean people.

Risk Factors
People with type 2 diabetes often have no symptoms, and their condition is detected only when a routine exam reveals high levels of glucose in their blood. Occasionally, however, a person with type 2 diabetes may experience

symptoms listed below, which tend to appear slowly over time.

⇒ Numbness or burning sensation of feet, ankles, and legs
⇒ Blurred or poor vision
⇒ Impotence
⇒ Fatigue
⇒ Poor wound healing

In some cases, symptoms may mimic type 1 diabetes and appear more abruptly, such as.

⇒ Excessive urination and thirst
⇒ Yeast infections
⇒ Whole body itching
⇒ Coma – in severe cases, high blood glucose may affect water distribution in brain cells, causing a state of deep unconsciousness, or coma.

FAMILY HISTORY OF TYPE 2 DIABETES

A quarter to one third of all individuals with type 2 diabetes have a family history of the condition.

⇒ Age older than 45 years
⇒ Excess body fat, particularly around the waist
⇒ Sedentary lifestyle and high-fat, high-calorie diet
⇒ Abnormal levels of cholesterol or triglycerides in blood
⇒ High blood pressure
⇒ History of gestational diabetes or polycystic ovarian syndrome, a hormonal disorder that causes women to have irregular or no menstruation

⇒ African American, Hispanic American, or Native American, particularly Pima tribe in Arizona descent

⇒ Low birth weight or a mother's malnutrition in pregnancy (this may cause metabolic disturbances in a fetus that lead to diabetes later in the child's life

⇒ Depression is associated with a 60% increased risk of type 2 diabetes

DIAGNOSIS

According to the American Diabetes Association, all pregnant women should be screened for gestational diabetes during their third trimester. People who are 45 years or older should have their blood glucose levels checked every 3 years. Those who have a high risk of developing diabetes, such as people with a family history of the disease, should be tested more often.

Different types of tests are used to diagnose diabetes. Random plasma glucose level, fasting plasma glucose level, and oral glucose tolerance test.

If the fasting glucose level is 100 to 125 mg/dL, the individual has a form of pre-diabetes called impaired fasting glucose (IFG), meaning that the individual is more likely to develop type 2 diabetes but does not have the condition yet. A level of 126 mg/dL or above, confirmed by repeating the test on another day, means that the individual has diabetes. The best test to find out if an individual's blood sugar is under control over time it to test every three months for insulin-treated people especially during treatment changes, or when blood glucose is elevated. For stable people, they should be tested at least twice per year. Studies have reported that there is a 10%

decrease in relative risk of microvascular complications, injuries to the small blood vessels throughout the body, such as diabetic nephropathy, kidney disease, or diabetic neuropathy, nerve damage, for every 1% reduction in haemoglobin A1c. Many nutritionally oriented physicians look for a much lower A1c as the goal for their patients.

Regular testing tells you how well your diet, medication, and exercise are working together to control your diabetes. Going for counselling with a Nutritionist can also be an integral part of preventive Care.

Considerable evidence from population-based studies suggests that type 2 diabetes is highly preventable, particularly through exercise and weight management. Individuals who are physically inactive or overweight are much more likely to develop type 2 diabetes. Similarly, people who move from a non-Westernized country to a Westernized country, such as the United States, where more people are overweight and live sedentary lives, increase their risk for type 2 diabetes. You do not need vigorous physical activity to lower your risk of diabetes; moderate, regular exercise, such as walking for 30 minutes most days of the week, is enough. In conclusion, general lifestyle changes are highly recommended to treat diabetes may help prevent the condition as well.

TREATMENT APPROACH

The goal of diabetes treatment is to achieve and maintain healthy blood glucose levels. A major study called the Diabetes Control and Complications Trial (DCCT) found that people with diabetes who kept their blood glucose levels close to normal reduced their risk of developing major complications from the condition.

People with diabetes can use the following therapies to help manage their blood glucose levels and to prevent complications.

⇒ Lifestyle changes, such as a well-balanced diet and regular exercise
⇒ Medications, particularly insulin for individuals with type 1 diabetes and some people with type 2 diabetes
⇒ Supplements, including fiber and chromium
⇒ Relaxation techniques
⇒ Acupuncture for pain from nerve damage

LIFESTYLE

People with diabetes can improve significantly from lifestyle changes, particularly diet and exercise. People with type 2 diabetes may even eliminate the need for medications when they make appropriate lifestyle changes.

DIET

The ADA recommends that people with diabetes consume a healthy, low-fat diet, rich in grains, fruits, and vegetables. A healthy diet typically includes 10 to 20% of daily calories from protein, such as poultry, fish, dairy, and vegetable sources. People with diabetes who also have kidney disease should work with their health care providers to limit protein intake to 10% of daily calories. A low-fat diet typically includes 30% or less of daily calories from fat, less than 10% from saturated fats and up to 10% from polyunsaturated fats, such as fats from fish.

Carbohydrates tend to have the greatest effect on blood glucose. The balance between the amount of carbohydrate eaten and the available insulin determines how much the blood glucose level goes up after meals or snacks. To help control blood glucose, people should watch how many carbohydrate servings they eat each day. Foods that contain a high amount of carbohydrates include grains, pasta, and rice; breads, crackers, and cereals; starchy vegetables, including potatoes, corn, peas, and winter squash; legumes such as beans, peas, and lentils; fruits and fruit juices; milk and yogurt; and sweets and desserts. Non-starchy vegetables, such as spinach, kale, broccoli, salad greens, and green beans, are very low in carbohydrates. Carbohydrate counting can ensure that the right amount of carbohydrate is eaten at each meal and snack. A nutritionist can help each person work out a dietary plan that is right for them.

In addition, weight loss should be part of the plan for those with type 2 diabetes. Moderate weight loss achieved by reducing calories by 250 to 500 per day and exercising regularly, controls not only blood sugars, but also blood pressure and cholesterol. People with diabetes who eat healthy, well-balanced diets do not necessarily need to take extra vitamins or minerals to treat their condition.

EXERCISE

Exercise plays an important role in both the prevention and management of diabetes because it lowers blood sugar and helps insulin work more efficiently in the body. Exercise also enhances cardiovascular fitness by improving blood flow and increasing the heart's pumping power, promoting weight loss and the lowering of blood pressure. However, exercise has the most value when it's done regularly, at least 3 to 4 sessions per week for 30 to 60 minutes per session. As little as 20 minutes of walking, 3 times a week, has proven to have beneficial effects. People with type 2 diabetes who exercise regularly have been shown to lose weight and gained better control over their blood pressure, thereby reducing their risk for cardiovascular disease, which is a major complication of diabetes. Studies have also shown that people with type 1 diabetes who exercise regularly reduce their need for insulin injections.

Despite the benefits of exercise, many people have difficulty sticking with an exercise program for a long period of time. Health care providers and fitness instructors can help develop motivational routines and strategies that may help to improve adherence to such routines. Anyone with long-standing diabetes should have a thorough screening before starting an exercise program and receive careful monitoring from a doctor.

MEDICATIONS

Medications for diabetes must always be used in combination with lifestyle changes, particularly diet and exercise, to improve the symptoms of diabetes. Medications include insulin, oral sulfonylureas, like glimepiride, glyburide, and tolazamide, biguanides, Metformin, alpha-glucosidase inhibitors, such as acarbose, thiazolidinediones, such as rosiglitazone and meglitinides, including repaglinide and nateglinide.

A new agent in the fight against diabetes, exenatide, Byetta, is an injectable drug that reduces the level of sugar in the blood. In clinical studies, patients treated with exenatide achieved lower blood glucose levels and lost weight. Exenatide was approved by the U.S. Food and Drug Administration in May 2005.

NUTRITION AND DIETARY SUPPLEMENTS
A lot of research has been conducted on the relationship between diabetes and specific nutrients and dietary supplements. Dietary supplements may increase the effects of blood sugar-lowering medications, including insulin. When considering the use of supplements or making dietary changes, be sure to discuss these changes with your health care provider to ensure safety and appropriateness.

SUPPLEMENTS WITH BLOOD SUGAR LOWERING EFFECTS
Chromium – Found in a variety of foods and supplements, including liver, brewer's yeast, cheese, meats, fish, fruits, vegetables, and whole grains, chromium appears to enhance the body's sensitivity to insulin. Researchers believe that chromium helps insulin pull glucose from the bloodstream into the cells for energy. The benefit of chromium supplements for diabetes has been studied and debated for years.

While some studies show no beneficial effects of chromium use for people with diabetes, other studies have shown that chromium supplements may reduce blood glucose levels in individuals with type 2 diabetes and reduce the need for insulin in those with type 1 diabetes.

The National Research Council estimates that intakes of 50 to 200 mcg per day are safe and effective. Clinical studies showing improved blood sugar control for those with diabetes have used doses of chromium picolinate ranging from 200 to 1,000 mcg per day. However, until human studies of long-term safety are conducted with higher doses, it is best to use 200 mcg or less per day. Chromium may interact negatively with insulin and thyroid medicines.

Magnesium – Several clinical studies have demonstrated a strong association between low levels of magnesium in the blood and type 2 diabetes. However, researchers are still unclear about the cause and effect in that association. They are investigating whether low magnesium levels worsen blood sugar control in people with type 2 diabetes or whether diabetes causes magnesium deficiencies. Some experts believe that low magnesium levels worsen blood sugar control and that foods rich in magnesium, such as whole grains, green leafy vegetables, bananas, legumes, nuts, and seeds, or magnesium supplements may promote healthy blood glucose levels.

Some studies do suggest that taking magnesium supplements may improve the action of insulin and decrease blood sugar levels, particularly in the elderly. People with severe heart disease or kidney disease should not take magnesium supplements. People with diabetes should talk with their health care provider about whether it's safe and appropriate to take magnesium supplements. Magnesium can interact negatively with some medications. Magnesium may lower blood pressure and cardiac output, and potentially interact with some cardiac medications but excessive amounts of magnesium can cause diarrhoea.

Fiber – Studies suggest that a high-fiber diet may help.

⇒ Prevent development of type 2 diabetes

⇒ Lower average glucose and insulin levels in people who already have type 2 diabetes

⇒ Improve cholesterol and triglyceride levels in those with diabetes

In a large-scale study of nurses in the United States, women who consumed the most whole grain foods in their diets were nearly 40% less likely to develop diabetes than women who consumed the least. People with irritable bowel syndrome, inflammatory bowel disease, or other digestive issues should speak with their doctor before adding fiber to their diet.

Studies have also shown that cholesterol levels improved in people with type 2 diabetes after they took supplements of a soluble fiber known as psyllium, Plantago psyllium. Also, Beta-glucan is a soluble fiber derived from the cell walls of algae, bacteria, fungi, yeast, and plants. It is commonly used for its cholesterol-lowering effects. There are several human trials supporting the use of beta-glucan for glycaemic, blood sugar, control.

Vanadium – Vanadium is an essential trace mineral present in the soil and in many foods. It appears to mimic the action of insulin and, in a number of human studies, vanadyl sulphate, a form of vanadium, has increased insulin sensitivity in those with type 2 diabetes. Some other studies suggest that it may lower blood glucose to normal levels, thus reducing the need for insulin in people with diabetes. One preliminary clinical study found that people with diabetes using insulin who were given vanadium were able to lower their dose of insulin. Vanadium may slow blood clotting, so people who take blood-thinning medication such as warfarin, Coumadin, and aspirin should check with their doctor before adding vanadium supplements to their regimen. People with a history of kidney issues should speak with their doctor before using vanadium supplements.

Melatonin – Melatonin is a natural hormone secreted in the brain and studies link low melatonin secretion with an increased risk of developing type 2 diabetes. Melatonin can cause sleepiness and potentially interact with some psychiatric medications and medications used to treat insomnia.

Antioxidants - such as beta-carotene and vitamin C are scavengers of free radicals, which are unstable and potentially damaging molecules generated by normal chemical reactions in the body. Free radicals are unstable because they lack one electron and, in their attempt, to replace this missing electron, the free radical molecules react with neighbouring molecules in a process called oxidation. Some clinical studies suggest that people with diabetes have elevated levels of free radicals and lower levels of antioxidants.

Preliminary clinical studies show that the following antioxidants may improve diabetes by returning blood glucose levels to the normal range and reduce the risk of associated complications.

⇒ Vitamin E
⇒ Selenium
⇒ Zinc
⇒ Quercetin
⇒ Lignaris

Two additional substances that show preliminary evidence to possibly help control blood sugar include.

⇒ Biotin, a B-complex vitamin, possibly helpful for type 2 diabetes; brewer's yeast is a good source of biotin
⇒ Vitamin B6, possibly helpful for both type 1 and type 2 diabetes

SUPPLEMENTS WITH CARDIOVASCULAR EFFECTS

Since insulin resistance is often associated with cardiovascular disease, people with diabetes may benefit from nutrients that help manage elevated blood lipid levels, high blood pressure, or heart failure. Although the following supplements have been shown to improve cardiovascular health, there is some concern that they may raise blood glucose levels, and they may interact with certain medications. People with diabetes interested in trying the following supplements should first consult with their health care providers.

⇒ Coenzyme Q10, CoQ10
⇒ Niacin
⇒ Omega-3 fatty acids

Although clinical studies have not shown that either CoQ10 or omega-3 fatty acid supplements raise blood sugar levels, people with diabetes should discuss the safety and appropriateness of using these, or any supplements, with their health care provider or pharmacist, particularly if they are taking other medications. CoQ10 can potentially increase the clotting tendency of blood while omega-3 fatty acids can potentially decrease it. Niacin in certain amounts can potentially damage the liver. Work with your physician to find the types and amounts of supplements that are right for you.

In addition, the following antioxidants have been shown to improve cholesterol levels in people with type 2 diabetes. Work with your doctor to see if these are appropriate for you as they can potentially interact with other medications and may potentially worsen other medical conditions.

⟹ Beta-carotene
⟹ Vitamin C (1000 mg per day)
⟹ Vitamin E (800 IU per day)

Several clinical studies have also found that elevated manganese levels may help protect against LDL oxidation, which is a process that contributes to the development of plaque in the arteries.

HERBS

People have long used plant-based medicines in the treatment of diabetes. For instance, the plant extract guanidine, which lowers blood glucose, prompted the development and use of biguanides, a commonly used oral medication for diabetes. Other herbs may have a role in the management or prevention of diabetes.

Always talk to your health care provider about any herbs you consider using. Some herbs may interact with medications, and some may lower your blood sugar. When combined with blood sugar-lowering medications, some herbs can bring your blood sugar to a dangerously low level.

Herbs that may have a role in the management or prevention of diabetes include.

Bitter melon - Momordica charantia. Bitter melon has traditionally been used as a remedy for lowering blood glucose in patients with diabetes. Preliminary clinical studies have indicated that bitter melon may decrease serum glucose levels. Bitter melon can be extremely dangerous to take when pregnant.

Fenugreek seeds - Trigonella foenum graecum. Fenugreek seeds, a spice found in many curry preparations, are high in fiber and have been shown to regulate glucose and improve lipid levels in humans. In other studies of people with either type 1 or type 2 diabetes, fenugreek seed powder lowered blood glucose and improved levels of blood cholesterol and triglycerides, among other beneficial effects. Fenugreek may interact with blood-thinning medications, such as warfarin, Coumadin.

Gymnema - Gymnema sylvestre. Preliminary human research reports that gymnema may be beneficial in patients with type 1 or type 2 diabetes when it is added to diabetes drugs being taken by mouth or to insulin. Gymnema may alter the ability to detect sweet tastes.

Cinnamon - Cinnamomum zeylanicum. In a clinical study of people with type 2 diabetes, intake of 1, 3, or 6 grams of cinnamon per day reduced glucose, triglyceride, LDL cholesterol, and total cholesterol levels and because some other clinical studies have found similar results, experts claim that cinnamon may play an important role in regulating blood sugar in people with diabetes.

American ginseng - Panax quinquefolium. Although both Asian, Panax ginseng and American Panax quinquefolium, ginseng appear to lower blood glucose levels, only American ginseng has been studied scientifically. Several clinical studies report a blood sugar-lowering effect of American ginseng, Panax quinquefolium in individuals with type 2 diabetes, both on fasting blood glucose and on postprandial glucose levels.

One clinical study found that people with type 2 diabetes who take American ginseng before or together with a glucose meal experience a reduction in glucose levels after they consume the meal. American ginseng may not be appropriate for people with auto immune disease, and may interact with several medications, including blood-thinning medications, such as warfarin, Coumadin, among others. People with a history of hormone-sensitive cancers should only use ginseng under the guidance of their physician.

ACUPUNCTURE

Some researchers speculate that acupuncture may trigger the release of natural painkillers and reduce the debilitating symptoms of a complication of diabetes known as neuropathy, nerve damage. In one clinical study of people with diabetes suffering from chronic, painful neuropathy, acupuncture reduced pain and improved sleep in 77% of the participants and eliminated the need for pain medications in 32% of the participants. Given these findings, acupuncture may be a reasonable option for people with diabetes who have neuropathy, and either find no symptom relief, or develop side effects from conventional drug treatment.

MIND-BODY MEDICINE

Stressful life events can worsen diabetes in several ways. For example, stress stimulates the nervous and endocrine systems in ways that increase blood glucose levels and disrupt healthful behaviors and increasing the chances that an individual may consume excess calories and limit his or her physical activity, a pattern that leads to elevated blood glucose.

It makes sense, then, to consider stress management as part of the treatment and prevention of diabetes. Clinical studies have reported that people with diabetes who participate in biofeedback sessions, a technique that increases awareness and control of the body's response to stress, are more likely to reach target blood glucose levels than those who do not receive biofeedback. Although other studies have produced conflicting results, researchers and clinicians agree that long-term stress is likely to worsen diabetes and that biofeedback, tai chi, yoga, and other forms of relaxation may help motivate people with diabetes to change their habits to manage their condition.

PREGNANCY

Women of child-bearing age who have diabetes should consult an endocrine specialist about the benefits of managing glucose levels before trying to conceive.

About 4% of all pregnant women in the United States are diagnosed with gestational diabetes. Risk factors for developing diabetes while pregnant include.

⇒ Modest weight gain prior to pregnancy of 11 to 22 pounds or more

$\Rightarrow$ Family history of diabetes

$\Rightarrow$ Tobacco use

$\Rightarrow$ African American, Hispanic American, or Asian ancestry

$\Rightarrow$ Age older than 50 at conception

Gestational diabetes is high blood glucose that develops at any time during pregnancy in a woman who does not have diabetes. Four percent of all pregnant women develop gestational diabetes. Although it usually disappears after delivery, the mother is at increased risk of developing type 2 diabetes later in life.

Normalizing glucose levels in women with gestational diabetes reduces their risk of complications, such as having an overweight baby, birth trauma, or the need for caesarean section. If the mother's glucose levels are uncontrolled, an infant can be stillborn or suffer from complications, including defects of the brain or central nervous system, an abnormally large body or organs, heart or kidney abnormalities, asphyxia, respiratory distress, and heart failure.

If dietary restrictions fail to improve glucose levels, a woman with gestational diabetes may need insulin. Women should not take oral diabetes medications during pregnancy. Women who develop gestational diabetes may experience the condition again in subsequent pregnancies.

Depressive symptoms are associated with an increased risk of diabetes. The association can't be explained by the use of antidepressant drugs or being overweight. Depression is an important risk factor for diabetes.

PROGNOSIS AND COMPLICATIONS

People who maintain tight control over their blood glucose levels can prevent or delay the development of long-term complications from diabetes. Type 1 diabetes generally has more complications than type 2 diabetes.

Long-term complications of diabetes may include.

⇒ Heart disease and stroke
⇒ Vision loss and blindness
⇒ Kidney disease
⇒ Neuropathy, nerve damage
⇒ Foot ulcers and infections
⇒ Skin problems, including bruising, dryness, itching, hair loss, warts, gangrene, tissue death, and skin ulcers

Chapter 9

Blood Pressure

Blood pressure (BP), sometimes referred to as arterial blood pressure, is the pressure exerted by circulating blood upon the walls of blood vessels. During each heartbeat, blood pressure varies between a maximum, systolic and a minimum, diastolic pressure. The blood pressure in the circulation is principally due to the pumping action of the heart.

⇒ Systolic - Systole is an ancient medical term first understood as a gathering of blood and later contraction of the heart. More recently it is understood as a force that drives blood out of the heart. It is the contraction of the left ventricle.

⇒ Diastolic – Diastole means dilation, it is the period of time when the heart refills with blood after systolic contraction.

Cardiac Cycle – Heartbeat

The cardiac cycle refers to a complete heartbeat from its generation to the beginning of the next beat, and so includes the diastole the systole and the intervening pause. The frequency of the cardiac cycle is described by the heart rate, which is typically expressed as beats per minute. Each beat of the heart involves five major stages.

⇒ Systolic

$\Rightarrow$ Diastolic

$\Rightarrow$ Isovolumic contraction

$\Rightarrow$ ventricular ejection

$\Rightarrow$ Isovolumic relaxation time

HEART RATE

Heart rate is the speed of the heartbeat, specifically the number of heartbeats per unit of time. The heart rate is typically expressed as beats per minute (bpm). The heart rate can vary according to the body's physical needs, including the need to absorb oxygen and excrete carbon dioxide. Activities that can provoke change include physical exercise, sleep, anxiety, stress, illness, ingesting, and drugs.

$\Rightarrow$ The normal human heart rate ranges from 60–100 bpm.

$\Rightarrow$ Bradycardia is a slow heart rate, defined as below 60 bpm.

$\Rightarrow$ Tachycardia is a fast heart rate, defined as above 100 bpm at rest.

$\Rightarrow$ When the heart is not beating in a regular pattern, this is referred to as an arrhythmia. These abnormalities of heart rate sometimes, but not always, indicate disease.

STROKE VOLUME

Stroke volume (SV) is the volume of blood pumped from one ventricle of the heart with each beat. Men, on average, have higher stroke volumes than women due to the larger size of their hearts. Aerobic exercise training may also increase stroke volume, which frequently results in a lower (resting) heart rate.

Cardiac Output

Cardiac output is the volume of blood being pumped by the heart, in particular by a left or right ventricle in the time interval of one minute. An average resting cardiac output would be 5.6 L/min for a human male and 4.9 L/min for a female.

Heart Rate During Exercise

The heart's blood flow increases by about four or five times from that of its resting state. Your body does this by increasing the rate of your heartbeat and the amount of blood that comes through the heart and goes out to the rest of the body. This increases the amount of blood returned to the heart venous return, which increases the stroke volume by about 30 to 40 percent. When the heart is pumping at full force, the cardiac output is about 20-25 litres per minute. As the lungs absorb more oxygen and the blood flow to the muscles increases, your muscles and body have more oxygen. When you begin to exercise, your heart rate increases rapidly in proportion to your exercise intensity.

Hypertrophy of Left Ventricle

Left ventricular hypertrophy (LVH) is the thickening of the myocardium (muscle) of the left ventricle of the heart. While ventricular hypertrophy occurs naturally as a reaction to over training aerobic exercise and strength training, it is most frequently referred to as a pathological reaction to cardiovascular disease, or high blood pressure.

While LVH itself is not a disease, it is usually a marker for disease involving the heart, primary disease of the muscle of the heart that cause LVH are known as hypertrophic cardiomyopathies, which can lead into heart failure.

Chapter 10

Gluten Sensitivity

Why do you feel fat and bloated after eating bread?

Gluten is a protein found in foods processed in wheat and consists of 80% protein that is found mainly in carbohydrates such as: wheat, barley and rye. Gluten is what makes dough doughy, it is responsible for elasticity of the dough. When the yeast is put into the dough the gluten molecules form a network of long chains that give dough its elasticity. Yeast jump starts and ferments the dough causing it to rise.

Gluten is made up of two parts both of which are starches. Glutenin and gliadin, the white powdery stuff you see on potatoes. This is what causes problems to people who suffer from gastrointestinal diseases because their digestive tract is not able to digest the gasses that are created from starchy carbohydrates.

The protein from glutenin in grits or oats like oatmeal, is a little different and therefore some people who suffer from celiac disease can eat them without a problem. When you use whole-wheat flour, gluten is what makes the bread heavy and dense. Gluten flours like from rye and spelt contain gluten in smaller quantities and comprise mainly of different types of proteins. Because of this, the impact of glutenin on your digestive tract is easier to process and digest.

Symptoms of gluten sensitivity include bloating, abdominal discomfort or pain, constipation and diarrhoea. There may be symptoms including muscular disturbances and bone or joint pain.

If you feel you may be sensitive to gluten, then you could test yourself by trying to live gluten-free for 2 weeks and see if your symptoms have gone, or you can do an endoscopic biopsy that can check your sensitivity with 100% accuracy.

The only way to treat gluten sensitivity right now is a gluten free diet, this gives your intestines a chance to heal and prevent more serious diseases from developing. You will have to read food labels really carefully and make sure it is written gluten-free. In some countries, gluten-free products are available on prescription and may be reimbursed by health insurance plans.

Chapter 11

Gastrointestinal Diseases

The importance of taking care of yourself.

Gastrointestinal diseases are referring to all diseases involving the gastrointestinal tract, such as the oesophagus, stomach, small intestine, large intestine and rectum. The digestion helper organs are the liver, gallbladder, and pancreas.

Stomach disease like inflammation or infection of the stomach is called gastritis, but when it involves other parts of the gastrointestinal tract it is then called gastroenteritis. When dealing with a chronic state, this means that several diseases are included: atrophic gastritis, pyloric stenosis, and gastric cancer. Gastric ulceration erodes the gastric mucosa which are the stomach mucus you develop to digest your food.

This is supposed to protect the tissue lining of the stomach from the stomach acids. Helicobacter pylori can be the culprit in causing gastric ulcers, so if you have any problems please deal with them immediately to prevent the illness from changing into a chronic disease.

The small and large intestines may be affected by any of the following infectious, autoimmune, or physiological conditions. Acute conditions affecting the bowels include infectious diarrhoea and mesenteric ischemia which is basically an inflammation of the small intestine due to a lack of blood supply. Some of the causes of constipation may be because of very hard stool or a bowel obstruction, but this may also be caused by the ileum which is the last section of the small intestine.

⇒ IBD – Inflammatory bowel disease is a condition whose origin is unknown. It may be classified as either Crohn's disease or ulcerative colitis, which is diagnosed only after Crohn's disease or ulcerative colitis have been ruled out.

⇒ IBS – Irritable bowel syndrome affects the intestines and other parts of the gastrointestinal tract by aggravating the lining of the digestive tract. Other causes of this illness are intestinal pseudo obstruction, and necrotizing enterocolitis.

⇒ IBD – Inflammatory bowel disease – Crohn's and Colitis

These are gastrointestinal diseases, and they are called diseases because they are recurring inflammations that occur in specific areas in the gut with a wide range of clinical symptoms.

Crohn's – known for its inflammatory ulcers on all of the lining and sub layer lining of the colon. People suffering with Crohn's disease have a high risk of developing partial ulcers. In 1932 Crohn and his colleagues localized the disease to mainly the ileum, which is the last section of the small intestine, but the disease can also develop along the mouth, oesophagus, stomach, duodenum, ileum and colon. Crohn's disease is often involved in the colon.

Colitis – ulcerative colitis is mostly limited to the lining of the colon and endometrial and its sub layer. This disease is diagnosed by the extent of its involvement which depends on how far up the colon the disease reaches. Ulcerative colitis is also associated with a general inflammatory process that typically affects many parts of the body.

Sometimes painful arthritic knees can be initial signs of the disease. It is also known as an extra-intestinal symptom. This can be seen in teenagers and adults alike though the presence of the disease may not be confirmed immediately, usually not diagnosed until the intestinal problems start showing up. Colitis is also always involved in the colon.

In rare cases of the condition, there are situations that can occur with colitis that it can be involved throughout all intestines, causing a reflux of acids to flare upwards, and so in both diseases there may be changes also in the small intestine.

People who suffer with Crohn's often have relatives who suffer from ulcerative colitis and vice versa. Both are clinically and pathologically similar diseases. From an epidemiological perspective, there are similarities that connect this disease, such as age, race, sex, and geographic regions.

Both diseases have similar manifestations outside the intestines.

Both diseases have an increased risk of malignancy in the colon.

CROHN'S

Characterized by chronic diarrhoea accompanied by abdominal pain, intermittent seizures, fever, low and lower right quadrant pain of the abdomen.

Anorexia, weight loss, flatulence, bloating, weakness and discomfort.

Sensitive stomach accompanied with the feeling of a lump in the abdomen.

ULCERATIVE COLITIS

⇒ Bloody diarrhoea accompanied by abdominal pain.
⇒ Tenderness in the abdomen, weight loss, fever.
⇒ Anal stimulation, fissures, haemorrhoids, fistulas and abscesses may be detected in a rectal examination.

CAUSES

IBD can occur at any age but usually appears between the ages of 25-35

⇒ More women suffer from the disease than men
⇒ Genetic tendency
⇒ Race
⇒ Dietary factors
⇒ Infectious factors
⇒ Response after trauma

IBD does not have a genetic marker that is predictive, but there is some genetic predisposition to factors that suggest a genetic predisposition. Prevalent among whites versus blacks, Jews versus non-Jews. 15%-40% of cases show that several people in one family suffer with colitis and Crohn's.

Infectious factors there are many factors involved in the speculation of which microorganisms' cause Crohn's and colitis. IBD Research of CMV, Cytomegalovirus which a virus related to herpes and EBV, Epstein-Barr virus, better known as Mono, shows that infections in the stomach such as Aeromonas, hydrophilic bacteria or candida albicans can initiate and cause colitis.

Pseudomonas – this is also a bacterium that contains many species that can initiate and perpetuate colitis. www. pseudomonas.com – this website is a data base that can provide you with more information if you need it.

Anaerobic gut bacteria like Enteric – It is a gut flora, which is always present in the gut and is usually harmless. Gut flora consists of a network of microorganism species that live in the digestive tract of animals and is the largest reservoir of human flora.

Crohn's is also associated measles. There is evidence that measles virus infection in early life may cause a tendency to develop Crohn's disease.

Antibiotics and Crohn's disease are linked in several cases in the U.S. and is on the rise since the increase in the multi ingestion of antibiotics. Researcher's conclusions are that the integral component that causes intestinal toxins in the flora is infection. The gut begins to produce toxic immunostimulants that become invasive because of sub-lethal doses of antibiotics, increasing the production of toxins in organisms in the gut. The bacteria do not get affected by these lethal doses of antibiotics, but their reaction is the adaption and strengthening of even more harmful bacteria. This weakens your immune mechanisms and also indicates that you may have an immune disorder, either primary or secondary.

DIETARY FACTORS

As you know, this disease is prevalent in all countries with Western diets and is increasing, compared to cultures that eat "primitive" diets and less industrialized diets, which have very few cases of Crohn's. Studies show that in patients who suffer with Crohn's, their diet prior to the outbreak of the disease included refined sugars and very little fibre.

One study shows the high intake of cereal like cornflakes which is rich in simple carbohydrates and is extracted from common allergen corn.

In Japan, there is a link between Crohn's disease and the low consumption of omega 3 and omega 6.

An increase in consumption of preservatives that include materials like Carnigen, a product that stabilizes, has been shown to constitute a cause of inflammation.

There is a study that shows that a deficiency in zinc can cause inflammatory bowel disease.

A physical or emotional trauma can trigger an outbreak of the disease.

It has been shown that children of parents who are smokers are more vulnerable to develop the disease.

MEDICATION

- ⇒ Derivative of salicylic acid.
- ⇒ Steroids that block Arachidonic acid release.
- ⇒ Drugs that suppress the immune system.

There are some cases that need surgical removal of the lesion, but this does not ensure that a recurrence of the lesions in other parts of the digestive tract will not occur.

COMPLICATION RISKS DUE TO IBD

25% of IBD patients have systematic complications of the disease. It is common in adults with arthritis especially in the knees, ankles and wrists.

15% of IBD patients have cutaneous lesions manifestations, which are different types of skin rashes and wounds.

10% of patients have mouth ulcers.

3.7% of patients have liver disease which makes sense because of the high levels of toxins in the body. • Can be expressed in the eyes, inflammation of the sclera.

The presence of calcium deposits in the kidneys due to overactive thyroid, hyperthyroid.

Gallstones.

Problem in child development and development of sexual organs.

LOW NUTRIENT ABSORPTION DUE TO IBD

65-75% of patients suffer weight loss resulting from their IBD because of loss of appetite and diarrhoea.

There is also low absorption in patients who underwent surgical intervention.

Non-absorption of fat is very common, as a result of so many lost calories and loss of fat-soluble vitamins.

Mineral loss due to diarrhoea.

Involvement of ilium can lead to malabsorption of vitamins and bile acids.

Patients with fatty stools should suspect the loss of calcium and magnesium.

In IBD sufferers there is an increased secretion of the proteins into the cavity of the intestines.

It is very typical in patients to have a decrease of plasma proteins.

Chronic blood loss can lead to iron deficiency.

NUTRITIONAL THERAPY

Dietary elimination – especially of wheat and dairy products.

Remove other allergens such as peanuts, tree nuts, shellfish, fish and soy and their derivatives.

Treatment should be based on complex carbohydrates and gluten-free products.

If the patient suffers from a deficiency of bile salts, it is best to consume fatty acids that are mono-unsaturated like olive oil and avocado.

Increase your intake of orange vegetables, a zinc deficiency will cause a decline of carotenes.

During a diarrhoea attack, do not consume fibre, only after, and then you should only eat water soluble fibres. They attract water and form a gel, which slows down digestion. Sources of soluble fibre, oatmeal, oat cereal, lentils, apples, oranges, pears, oat bran, strawberries, nuts, flaxseeds, beans, dried peas, blueberries, psyllium, cucumbers, celery, and carrots.

SUPPLEMENTS THAT CAN HELP

Zinc – deficiency is present in half of IBD patients. You may have symptoms such as a taste impairment or a decreased rehabilitation rate from injuries, decline in fertility, and dysfunction of the retina. The zinc injection has been shown to be ineffective since zinc is excreted in your urine. Zinc sulphate showed negative results but zinc Picolinate was found to be effective.

Magnesium – 200-400mg magnesium is advisable but because magnesium can cause diarrhoea, which is not what you want, some patients may need to receive it via injection.

Iron – In cases of anaemia you should take iron, preferably with vitamin C. It is best to take iron in liquid form.

Potassium – deficiency characterizes itself in diarrhoea diseases. Studies have shown that reinforcement of potassium in your diet reduces surgical complications.

Vitamin A – 20% of patients have low levels of retinol. There is a correlation between retinol during the disease and its effect on the mucous membranes. Yet long-term studies have not shown that vitamin A yields results. With certain people zinc addresses the problem because it is an essential metabolite protein conspirator.

Vitamin D – there is evidence that vitamin D is deficient in most people who suffer from IBD. It is worth taking because of its immunological affects, and because you want to prevent osteoporosis.

Vitamin E – Recommend that you take vitamin E because it slows down and inhibits leucocytes and oxidative damage.

Vitamin K – Deficiency of vitamin K can cause osteoporosis which is very common in IBD sufferers. Folic acid – 64% of patients are deficient in folic acid. A deficiency in folic acid affects and changes the structure of mucosal cells that change every 4 days. Patients with Crohn's have a genetic defect in the metabolism of folic acid and moreover, some drugs administered to treat IBD damage it too, so it is good to take folic acid. But take this with Vitamin B12 and not alone.

Vitamin B12 – Vitamin B12 is deficient in most people who had a part of their ileum removed. There is no absorption of vitamin B12 if the length of damage is 60cm or more.

Vitamin C – Because people who suffer from IBD consume a diet low in fruits and vegetables vitamin C is essential for preventing deficiency of vitamins and leukocytes. Vitamin C is crucial in the prevention of fistulas, so it is worthwhile taking.

Multivitamins – Since a lot of patients have a deficiency in various nutrients it is advisable to take multivitamins and minerals of high quality because of their antioxidant qualities to combat the high levels of oxidation and toxins that stress has released into the body.

Quercetin – Important for release of inflammatory mediators from mast cells, also known as healing cells, and lowers leucocytes levels.

HERBS

- ⇒ Althea – soothes mucous membranes
- ⇒ Echinacea – antibacterial
- ⇒ Hydrastis – inhibits the growth of bacteria
- ⇒ Phytolacca – heals ulcers

⇒ Comfrey – anti-inflammatory

⇒ Elm – Demulcent, a pain reliever, soothes

In a pot add cabbage powder and Niatzinamid

Probiotics – very important to repair the flora in your intestines by replacing harmful microbes for microbes that help us.

IBS – IRRITABLE BOWEL SYNDROME

Is a functional colon disorder without structural defects, the syndrome is characterized by a combination of the following symptoms.

⇒ Abdominal pain and alternation between constipation and diarrhoea

⇒ Excessive secretion of mucus from the colon

⇒ Symptoms of flatulence, nausea.

⇒ Anxiety or depression levels vary Splenic flexure syndrome is sometimes classified as sub irritable bowel syndrome

⇒ Gases in the colon leading to lower chest pain or in the left shoulder

⇒ Many patients with IBS suffer from an increase in sexual dysfunction

⇒ Fibromyalgia, urinary frequency, insomnia and headaches, Chronic fatigue

IBS tendency to increase and worsen and most common amongst.

⇒ Women – there are two women to every one man who tend to suffer from IBS.

- ⇒ People suffering with IBS reported mainly "excess flatulence."
- ⇒ Stomach noises, hiccups, uncontrolled gas emissions.
- ⇒ These effects significantly impair quality of life.

We all produce and hoard gas in our digestive system which we emit sub consciously approximately 600ml every day.

WHERE DOES THE GAS COME FROM?

About one-third is from swallowing air while drinking, talking or eating.

The greater part is formed from the breakdown of food components by intestinal bacteria.

Carbohydrates are the main ingredients broken down by bacteria, including.

Beans, cabbage, wheat, fructose, lactose, sorbitol and starch.

Fats and proteins produce less gas. IBS sufferers say they have a flat stomach in the morning which swells up by the evening, especially after meals. Some suffers say their stomach swells to the dimensions of pregnancy. There is no indication of IBS suffers to date having increased gas volume, only that their gut has a dysfunctional response to gasses. They have an excessive delay in emitting gasses which causes convulsive headaches and feeling swollen, whereas in healthy people the gas runs through their intestines. IBS suffers are more susceptible to a normal amount of gas, and their digestive tract reacts to it with pain, nausea and bulges.

DIAGNOSIS

IBS is diagnosed by ruling out other diseases.

⇒ Frequent and painful bowel movements, swelling, pain relief after the egestion, a nice way of saying going to the bathroom.
⇒ Faecal examination is necessary to rule out other things.
⇒ Evaluation of ESR.
⇒ If you suffer from a lot of diarrhoea you should check for celiac antibodies.
⇒ It is necessary to do a faecal occult blood test and Sigmoidoscopy in patients who are 50 and over.

A colonoscopy should be done in patients aged 50. Patients under the age of 50 should have a colonoscopy if they have the following symptoms.

⇒ Suffer from stress or lead a very fast paced lifestyle
⇒ People who use laxatives
⇒ Eat an unbalance diet
⇒ Drink excessive amounts of caffeine
⇒ Smokers
⇒ People who eat a lot of simple sugars
⇒ People who often suffer from IBS after gastrointestinal infections
⇒ Abnormal gut flora and Diabetes

THERAPEUTIC CONSIDERATIONS

Our approach to treat this is in three main ways, 1. Increasing dietary fibre. 2. You reduce food factors that causes intolerance, and 3. Relaxation. People who swallow air when eating, should make the effort of eating slowly and chew well.

⇒ Eat small meals.
⇒ Avoid chewing gum and drinking carbonated drinks.
⇒ Don't run around doing other things, and please don't eat when you are stressed. Sit and eat only when you are calm.
⇒ Eat dietary fibres.

If you suffer from constipation you will respond well to more fibre in your diet.

Fibre from fruits and vegetables are preferred, 30g fibre from vegetables and 10g of fibre from grains.

Guar Gum is a recommended fibre that has been hydrolysed, basically broken down.

If you suffer from diarrhoea it is best to eat cooked vegetables and in small amounts.

FOOD ALLERGIES

There are many studies that talk about food intolerance.

The most common food intolerance for between 40%-44% of IBS sufferers is dairy products, and cereal for between 40%-60% of IBS suffers.

IBS sufferers should be administered a hypoallergenic food diet and gradually weaned back onto normal food.

It is advisable to remove from your diet, citrus fruits, chocolate, caffeine, alcohol.

High levels of beans and sugar could cause IBS. When blood glucose levels rise rapidly the duodenum and the jejunum become toneless after this rapid glucose uptake.

This condition is very common in the U.S.

IBS is also connected with sensitivity to fructose as a sweetener.

Exercise is very important.

SUPPLEMENTS THAT CAN HELP

⇒ Herbs such as chamomile.
⇒ Verbena
⇒ Basswood, lime.

AROMATHERAPY

⇒ Peppermint oil – to soothe muscles.

You can either add to your bath or make a compress to hold on your abdomen, neroli, chamomile and lavender.

Bach flowers may relieve anxiety and stress.

LEAKED BOWEL SYNDROME

The primary function of a healthy gut lining is preventing the penetration of toxins and bacteria from entering the blood stream. this is the reason that there is a natural barrier consisting of epithelial, skin cells and tissue nodes, a disruption of which can lead to intestinal damage at the checkpoint, allowing passage of bacteria into the digestive tract.

Gastric Intrinsic Factors are proteins that contain carbohydrate chains attached to them. They protect the small intestine whose hosting contains internal factors that prevent the intrusions of environmental pathogens.

Typically, there is a passive resistance of the passage of very high potential toxins, so if the regulatory molecules will be affected by the bacterial toxins, cytokines hormones can alter the permeability of connective proteins.

The lymphatic system of the digestive tract prevents the passage of harmful molecules from the intestinal mucosa into the bloodstream. Immune cells consist of 40% of the mass and the intestine contains 25% of the gut mucosa.

This consists of two Defence mechanisms – the specific system consists of immunoglobulin and the non-specific system is very complex and consists of acid mucosa, digestive enzymes, flora levels and antibodies.

Dysfunction of the intestinal barrier can cause an immune deficiency which can then result in changes in the intestinal flora or indirect mucosal injury.

Normal intestinal micro flora "prevents settlement" of pathogens entering through intestinal walls. Changes in the bowel can impair its natural defences and encourage potential settlement of harmful bacterial strains.

Different mechanisms of bacteria and their toxins can change intestinal permeability. This is a normal function of the intestine to have some permeability, but also to maintain a barrier, whereby potentially harmful bacteria are prevented from leaving the intestine and migrating to the body.

Bacteria can secrete enzymes, for example, elastase and protease. They perform hydrolysis on the epithelial membrane, cell wall, thereby causing the separation of epithelial cells from the sides. Toxic bacteria and poisons can function either on or from within the membrane and damage the connective proteins' strength by connecting to their membrane receptors.

These are toxins that can prevent protein synthesis production and damage cell function and prevent cell growth. They can also change the composition of the lipid, fat membrane or create holes in the membrane which is the cell wall.

Since the intestinal mucosa plays a significant role in the immune system and absorption of nutrients, it has been associated with a variety of diseases and abnormal syndromes and intestinal permeability, which is a condition where the intestinal wall has been invaded.

LEAKY INTESTINE'S RELATED DISEASES

⇒ IBD inflammatory bowel disease
⇒ Ankylosing spondylitis that causes stiffness of vertebrae, and rheumatoid arthritis
⇒ Celiac disease and food allergies
⇒ Rheumatoid arthritis
⇒ Cancer and chemotherapy patients
⇒ Diabetes
⇒ Alcoholism
⇒ NSAIDS Non-steroidal anti-inflammatory drugs

IBD – Inflammatory bowel disease is typically an overreaction of the immune system of the gastrointestinal retrieval system. It is thought that the trigger is an intestinal barrier disorder that increases mucosal antigenic load.

Studies show that tests can detect intestinal permeability in patients with recurring Crohn's disease even during remission. Crohn's patients treated for intestinal permeability had a higher remission rate.

The Celiac disease's pathophysiology is the most diverse, ranging from patients with a lack of symptoms to other patients with severe symptoms such as diarrhoea and anaemia. Irrespective of the intensity of the disease doctors must treat all their celiac patients with a gluten-free diet to prevent complications of infertility and malignancy. There is a high percentage of intestinal permeability in patients with celiac disease who are not treated in contrast to patient who have been treated and can be rehabilitated in five months.

Food Allergies – Studies show excess reactivity causes oedema, and disruption of immunoglobulin Ig E, also known as type 1 hypersensitivity membrane, and the Ig G-type which controls infection in the body, causing a swift and progressive deterioration reaction. In vitro tests of both types showed an increase in the ability of large molecules to move spontaneously and actively, which indicates disruption of the mucosal barrier.

Diabetes – Studies show that diabetics, more common in type 1, suffer from mucosal dysfunction and because of which, they have an increased risk of developing intestinal permeability, as well as a gluten sensitivity.

Arthritis – Several studies have shown a correlation between various types of arthritis and increased intestinal permeability. It remains to be determined whether the correlation has arisen from the disease itself or from taking NSAIDS following treatment. It looks like Ankylosing spondylitis, osteoporosis patients have increased risk of intestinal permeability, but it cannot be determined if the permeability originates from the disease or from the drug therapy.

Alcoholism – Consumption of alcohol may cause or increase the risk of intestinal permeability disease, causing infections of the hepatic bile. Alcohol significantly increases intestinal permeability even two weeks after consuming alcohol.

FACTORS AFFECTING INTESTINAL PERMEABILITY

NSAIDS – cause intestinal permeability in 65% of people taking them. Most people develop intestinal permeability after taking them for a year.

Intestinal infection – contaminated food and drinks, stress and antibiotics, cause a wide range may of damage to the mucosal barrier.

Chemotherapy – there is increased risk of intestinal permeability during chemotherapy treatment, since the enterocytes, intestinal cells are rapidly dividing cells and are sensitive to chemotherapy. Bowel function returns to normal after two weeks of stopping treatment.

SYMPTOMS

⇒ Fatigue
⇒ Food intolerance
⇒ Abdominal pain
⇒ Diarrhoea
⇒ Rashes
⇒ Low tolerance for physical activity
⇒ Damage to memory and cognitive activity
⇒ Abdominal swelling

Diagnostic tests for intestinal leakage

Claude Andre – French researcher found non-invasive diagnostic testing for intestinal permeability. Andre's protocol was that each patient would receive 5g of sugars mannitol and lactulose. These sugars are excreted in the urine in 6 hours. The patient then gives a urine sample in the morning after 8 hours of fasting after taking the sugars. Mannitol, a simple sugar passively transported through intestinal walls, its average absorption is 14% of the portion taken. Lactulose, a disaccharide whose absorption is usually less than 1% was blocked by the intestine. 5. 6 hours later urine levels were measured. The average ratio of mannitol: lactulose is -0.03. A higher ratio indicates greater absorption of lactulose hence the leaky gut.

Supplements that can help

Glutamine – is an amino acid essential for the normality and quality of the mucosa. Basically, it balances the intestinal mucus to normal levels. Glutamine L rehabilitates and restores the function of the small intestine.

Probiotics – Lactobacillus Rhamnosus bacteria increases interferon gamma production which allows protection of the mucosa. Bifidobacterium lowers levels of interleukin to 1, 6 thus preventing damage to connective tissue proteins. Probiotics stimulates non-specific resistance of the pathogenic bacteria.

Fatty Acids – omega 3, test tube studies show that Eicosanoids which are derived from omega 3 fatty acids is a pro-inflammatory, so it is recommended to take Omega-3.

GLA – Gamma-Linoleic acid from evening primrose oil, administering GLA to treat the mucous membrane because it is a precursor, which means that it participates in a chemical reaction that produces prostaglandin E1.

Glucosamine – Protects mucous membranes from exposure to acids, very important for IBD sufferers. Studies shows it encourages a growth in Bifidobacterium and inhibits the growth of Candida in the intestine. In addition, it connects to the lectins in your diet and thus reduces the harmful impact on your intestines.

Digestive enzymes – are enzymes found in the digestive tract that help to digest food.

Vitamin C and bioflavonoids – strengthens your connective tissue.

NUTRITIONAL THERAPY

- ⇒ Hypoallergenic diet.
- ⇒ GLA containing oats.
- ⇒ Flaxseed oil contains Fatty Acid ALA alpha-linoleic acid.

CELIAC

In 1888 a British physician named Samuel Jones Gee described a strange health phenomenon in a child. Despite normal diet she had suffered from malnutrition, diarrhoea and weight loss. In those days, they did not know how to treat those children and eventually this shortened their lives.

Celiac patients were characterized as short, extremely thin, with a lack of subcutaneous fat and a bulging belly suggesting hunger and malnutrition, with chronic diarrhoea, fatty stools and delayed sexual development.

Celiac disease is a metabolic disorder, usually congenital, characterized as a inability to digest gluten-containing proteins. The disease causes malabsorption and defective structure of the small intestine mucosa.

Factors

Genetic background – 10% prevalence of first-degree relatives. The disease does not always develop in childhood, in 20% of cases the disease flares up after the age of 60 the disease could erupt after surgery, pregnancy, childbirth, viral infection and extreme stress situations. the gluten and its polypeptide derived gliadin that has not been through break down are the cause of the disease. Gluten is mainly found in wheat, barley, rye, oats and spelt.

Symptoms

- ⇒ Abdominal pain
- ⇒ Diarrhoea
- ⇒ Fatty stools
- ⇒ Weight loss
- ⇒ Deficiencies of vitamins and minerals
- ⇒ Usually develops lactose intolerance

Because the disease affects the walls of the small intestine, celiac patients suffer from significant nutritional deficiencies.

Diagnosis

A blood test for beta gliadin and a biopsy of the small intestine

Nutritional therapy, avoiding gluten for life

Avoid dairy products that contain lactose

Look out for concealed gluten-containing ingredients in foods

A diet rich in fruits and vegetables, legumes, seeds and nuts

If there is a delay in recovery other sensitivities should be checked for

SUPPLEMENTS

⇒ Zinc lozenges – for mucosal renewal, patients who were deficient in zinc had a delay in their recovery.
⇒ Digestive aids – lactase.
⇒ Multivitamin – make sure that it is gluten free.
⇒ Herbs – chamomile, it is gentle and suitable for all ages.

Research conducted at the University of Washington examined the prevalence of celiac and osteoporosis. The study found that the more severe celiac disease was, this made osteoporosis more severe too. Gluten-free diet treatment resulted in significant improvement in bone density.

Researchers concluded that the incidence of celiac disease in patients who suffered from osteoporosis is more common, and they recommend that all osteoporosis patients should also be tested for celiac.

ALLERGIES

IgE – immediate allergy

Allergies connected to IgE have extreme and swift reaction, less than 5% incidences. They develop quickly and can also be genetic. That means that there are specific tendencies that produce certain types of antibodies like IgE towards certain foods like for example celiac disease.

IgE antibody attaches to the antigen, specific allergen.

When there are enough antigens.

The antibodies cause the mast cells to release their granule contents, causing the release of chemical and inflammatory product from the body.

IgE type antibody is identified as an allergen whose source is in food connected to it. The antibody connects to the other side of the mast cell. When the problematic food is eaten the mast, cell sticks on to it and releases histamine that causes a variety of symptoms. These are all combat fields for allergic reactions of IgE type, skin, intestines, and respiratory system.

IgG – delayed allergy

IgG delayed allergic reaction is very common amongst children and one in every three people. It occurs when the immune system produces too many IgG antigens as an allergic reaction to food.

Instead of sticking to the mast cell like the IgE antigen, the IgG antigen connects directly to the food particles as they enter the blood stream causing their immobilization. IgG antibodies enter the blood stream and form an "immune complex" which rapidly increases in numbers. After this the immunization process gets into action and kicks in and sending phagocytes to swallow up the allergen.

This is a long process which is the reason why the symptoms don't appear right away. It could take between two hours to two days after eating the allergen food. For example, a migraine can appear two days after eating the food.

DIFFERENCES BETWEEN THE TYPES OF ALLERGIES

IgG ALLERGY

Affects children and adults

Reaction shows between 2 hours and 2 days

There are cases where symptoms appeared also between 3 to 7 days after eating food

Can be caused by 3 to 10 types of food with sensitive people, or even more

The symptoms don't appear right away, so it is not always easy to diagnose by oneself and stop eating it

Is caused by common food that most people are used to eating, and are specially craved

1 in 3 can suffer from these withdrawal symptoms

⇒ Delayed reaction is likely to affect all of the organs, fibres and systems of the body
⇒ Delayed reactions require advanced blood tests to localize the presence of the IgG antigen

IgE ALLERGY

Affects children and rarely adults

Symptoms appear immediately after eating

Exposure to 1 to 2 types of food

Even a small amount of the food causes a reaction

Can be caused by scarce foods

If stopped eating, you don't suffer from withdrawal symptoms

Immediate reaction affects mainly the skin, respiratory system and digestive system

Can be diagnosed by a skin graft

Allergies affect the whole body. These are symptoms that occur from head to foot,

- ⇒ Headache, migraine, fatigue
- ⇒ Depression, anxiety
- ⇒ Hyperactivity
- ⇒ Itchy eyes
- ⇒ Dark circles under eyes
- ⇒ Facial swelling
- ⇒ Cold and runny nose
- ⇒ Hay fever 66
- ⇒ Recurring mouth sores
- ⇒ Muscle cramp
- ⇒ Itchy skin
- ⇒ Eczema
- ⇒ Asthma or difficulty in breathing
- ⇒ Nauseous or vomiting
- ⇒ Ulcers in stomach, or duodenum

Diarrhoea, IBS, constipation, gassy stomach, swelling of stomach, water retention, Crohn's disease, and stomach pains

- ⇒ Joint pain
- ⇒ Inflammation of joints

⇒ Laryngeal, throaty

⇒ Enema, water retention

COMMON ALLERGAN FOODS

⇒ Cow's milk

⇒ Wheat

⇒ Yeast

⇒ Eggs

⇒ Soya

⇒ Walnuts

⇒ Corn

⇒ Oats

⇒ Lentils

⇒ Kiwi

⇒ Sesame

⇒ Nuts

⇒ Preservatives and food colourings

⇒ Fish

CAUSES OF ALLERGIES

⇒ Overload on the immune system

⇒ Early withdrawal from mother's milk

⇒ Permeability of the intestine, damage to intestines because of injury or inflammation and an imbalance in the flora

⇒ Genetic

⇒ Exaggerated craving for a certain food

⇒ Lacking in nutrition

NUTRITIONAL TREATMENT

⇒ Worthwhile to perform a liver cleanse

⇒ Circuit diet – every 4 days returning to the same food
⇒ Elimination diet – every 4 weeks add back omitted foods
⇒ Increase fruits and vegetables that contain oxidization, apples rich in quercetin
⇒ Advisable to eat organic food
⇒ Fatty acids like omega 3
⇒ Eat foods without gluten

SUPPLEMENTS THAT CAN HELP

⇒ Omega 3
⇒ Vitamin C – 1 to 2 grams
⇒ MSM – 1000-1600 micrograms
⇒ Zinc – 15 mg
⇒ Quercetin – 500 mg + Bromelain 125 mg + 250-300 micrograms Vitamin C – 3 times a day

Chapter 12

Fibromyalgia

Classified as a generalized muscular pain and fatigue.

Pain is the most prominent symptom of Fibromyalgia. Although it generally affects the entire body, it may start in just one region, such as the neck and shoulders which then spread to other areas over a period of time. Fibromyalgia is classified as a form of generalized muscular pain and fatigue. Therefore, it has been treated exactly as that since the initial diagnosis was developed years ago. But you now know through scientific research that the disease is actually a neurological condition that is caused by gradually increasing levels of inflammation in the body.

Inflammation will cause muscles to ache and burn, it will also cause muscles to spasm and develop the hallmark trigger points or tender points commonly associated with the diagnosis of Fibromyalgia.

2% of Americans suffer from Fibromyalgia, it manifests itself between the ages of 20-40. Fibromyalgia is often not diagnosed right away because most of its typical symptoms can be characterized and mistaken for other medical conditions. Fibromyalgia mainly affects muscles and connective tissues, which means that it may affect the Vascular tissues, which are heart muscles.

Fibromyalgia mainly affects the neck, shoulders, chest, lower back and hips. Since Fibromyalgia is only diagnosed after other diseases are ruled out, people suffer for a long time without and official diagnosis and treatment.

SYMPTOMS

Severe throbbing Pain which usually appears in all parts of the body, which it typically will start in one area and spread to other various areas of the body. Sometimes there are changes in the level of pain and location depending on time of day, activity level, weather changes and degree of stress. Humidity aggravates the disease also.

Fibromyalgia Patients always have some degree of pain accompanied with a constant feeling of flu symptoms. They suffer from Tender points around the lower lumbar vertebra. Second rib and around the upper part of the femur. Muscles at the base of skull, Upper back muscles, Middle of the knee joint. Muscles in the middle back, Sides of the elbow and at the bottom of the back

Patients suffer constant Fatigue and sleep disorders, in addition to their constant fatigue, they suffer lack of energy ranging from moderate to severe levels. Patients suffering from sleep disorders tend to wake up several times a night.

NERVOUS SYSTEM SYMPTOMS

Many patients suffer from mood swings and feel sad. Even though only 25% of patients suffer from clinical depression. Patients suffer from anxiety, difficulty in concentrating and performing simple mental tasks.

OTHER PROBLEMS

Other symptoms include Headaches but mainly due to muscular contraction.in the neck. Abdominal pain with a bloating sensation, they may also suffer diarrhoea and constipation with alternating spasms in the bladder. Their skin colour changes due to changes in temperature.

So now you see from this list of very unpleasant symptoms of Fibromyalgia, that are not consistent, how it is easy to not be able to diagnose it.

WHAT ARE ITS CAUSES?

- ⇒ Lowered immune system
- ⇒ Stress resulting from physical or mental trauma
- ⇒ Hypothyroidism
- ⇒ Candida or intestinal parasites
- ⇒ Chemical poisoning
- ⇒ Exposure to cold

DIAGNOSIS

As you explained that Symptoms for Fibromyalgia are diagnosed by ruling out other diseases. But these are typical symptoms that appear with Fibromyalgia, and as you learn more about this disease, you can recognise its widespread pain in all four quadrants of the body which lasts for at least 3 months.

Their pains are in sensitive areas of the body, more are severe in the morning and declines during the course of the day. The pain concentrates on specific points in the body without projecting to other areas.

TREATMENT

- ⇒ Relaxation techniques, guided meditation, stretching, yoga.

⇒ Nutritional therapy, eat every three hours to conserve energy

⇒ Vegetables, fruits, nuts, seeds.

⇒ Chicken, turkey and fish.

⇒ Avoid milk and dairy products.

⇒ Avoid caffeine.

SUPPLEMENTS THAT CAN HELP

⇒ Probiotics to improve digestive system

⇒ Q10

⇒ Vitamins B Complex

⇒ Omega 3

Chapter 13

Inflammatory Diseases

Distinguishing between two types of inflammations.

Long term inflammatory diseases if left untreated eventually start to damage different areas of the body, such as the brain, the nervous system, the digestive tract and the endocrine system. When these systems start to fail, you start to see classic signs and symptoms of the inflammatory diseases.

⇒ Fatigue, lethargy, decreased energy levels
⇒ Brain fog or fi bro fog
⇒ Headaches
⇒ Cold hands and feet
⇒ Insomnia
⇒ Digestive problems or IBS

Inflammation is the immune system's reaction against pathogens, injury or irritants. Inflammation is not an infection, even though an infection can cause an inflammation, but not all inflammation is infectious. Inflammation is essential for the survival of man because the reason there is an inflammation, is your body's attempt to protect you by removing damaging agents that have infiltrated your body and initiate a healing process. Let you distinguish between two types of inflammation.

ACUTE INFLAMMATION

This inflammation is an immediate response reaction controlled by the vascular cells and the immune system. This inflammation heals spontaneously and is generally short lived. It can last anywhere from minutes to several days.

GENERAL CAUSES

⇒ Bacteria
⇒ Virus
⇒ Fungus
⇒ Traumatic, Injuries
⇒ Infection

CHRONIC INFLAMMATION

This type of inflammation can continue for long periods of time, even weeks and in some cases years. Chronic inflammation may even develop after an acute inflammation or following an acute autoimmune disease.

If this inflammation is not regulated or treated properly and continues for a long period of time, there is a risk of the inflammation causing damage or injuring tissue and destroying adjacent tissues.

Chronic inflammation is a sign that there may be a serious disruption in the function of the bodily systems. So instead of protecting you or trying to heal us, the inflammation is causing you debilitating and excessive injuries and illnesses.

Chronic inflammation generates an immune response characterized by constant and excessive cytokines activity. More and more white blood cells move to the inflammation site. The body's Defence systems are now operating in surplus in an attempt to bring about healing. This uncontrolled process can initiate the activation of an inflammation, resulting in a devastating assault on the joints, organs or arteries and leading to the weakening and exhausting of the bodily systems.

EXAMPLES OF CONDITIONS THAT MAY BE CAUSED BY CHRONIC INFLAMMATION.

⇒ Arthritis
⇒ Allergies
⇒ Dermatitis
⇒ Chronic sinusitis
⇒ Liver disease
⇒ Bowel disease

Chronic Inflammation Terminologies and understanding how they affect your health is important in taking responsibility for your ability to maintain good health.

Cytokines – are a broad and loose category of small proteins licensed by vaccine cells. Their role is to mediate and regulate immune responses and inflammation. Cytokines are produced by the intrusion of the antigen to the body and are divided into several groups, chemokines, interferons, interleukins, and lymphokine.

Interleukin – a protein that belongs to the cytokines family and is secreted by leukocytes. They work as the signalling proteins. There exists up to 30 interleukins marked as IL. They adhere to a molecule on the cell surface sending signals to the cell, acting as a growth factor and play a role in suppressing the immune system.

IL interleukin-1 – cytokine which leads to the increase in body temperature and slows the virus or bacteria activity. Interleukin is associated with many inflammatory diseases particularly interleukin-1 like arthritis and Alzheimer's.

IL interleukin-6 – secreted by macrophages 6 and by other immune cells. Signalling to the immune system to produce antibodies. Abnormal production of IL-6 is associated with autoimmune disorders and allergies. Too much production accelerates pain and inflammation and causes certain immune cells to destroy the tissues, the organs and joints.

Histamine

A substance secreted by the body when the mast cells respond to an allergy reaction including asthma. Histamine is abundant in mast cells of the connective tissue, muscles, tendons, ligaments and muscle coating. It is secreted in response to injury or invasion of pathogens, causing the inflammation and expansion of blood vessels, which promotes pain and upper respiratory secretions. Histamine increases the permeability of blood vessels.

NF – kappa B protein is activated as part of the inflammatory response of the immune system to invasive organisms and damaged tissue and involved in cell division.

Prostaglandins

Prostaglandins are hormone-like lipids produced naturally in many tissues of the body from the dismantling of Arachidonic acid. They contribute to the correct running of gastrointestinal mucosa, platelets and kidneys, and are involved in the inflammatory response in the body and uterine contraction.

Prostaglandins promote pain, swelling and redness. Prostaglandins produced by CoX2 enzymes are inflammatory, increasing the intensity of pain, in contrast to CoX1 enzymes which participate in the healing process. TNF, tumour necrosis factor alpha, also involved in inflammation system, though its primary role is to regulate immune cells. When it is secreted it induces heat, fever and inflammation and also cell death. Large amounts of TNF are released in response to immune cells as a result of the inflammation.

C reactive protein – is a substance that is produced in the liver during the inflammatory response process. High levels of CRP raise the risk of heart disease, diabetes and cancer.

STAGES OF ACUTE INFLAMMATION
TRIGGER – THERE IS AN INVASION OF A FOREIGN BODY OR AN INJURY.

Phase 1 - bacteria or foreign object penetrates skin layer and enters the bloodstream and stimulates the immune system response.

ACTIVATE – GOES INTO ACTION.

Phase 2 - cytokines activated and released into the blood stream to alarm the problem.

MOBILIZE – ACTIVATION AND MOBILIZATION OF THE IMMUNE SYSTEM.

Phase 3 - cytokines secreted by immune cells migrate to location of the infection. Mast cells secrete histamine, to alert the occurrence of the injury and to increase blood flow to the damaged area, thus this creates redness, pain and swelling.

ERADICATE – NEUTRALIZING AND DESTROYING THE PATHOGEN.

Phase 4 - macrophages migrate to the scene of the injured tissue and the phagocyte engulfs the bacteria into the cell sinkhole. The waste from the defective cells is removed from the body using enzymes released by white blood cells.

REPAIR – HEALING.

Phase 5 - immune cells move into the affected area and while the area is being cleared, more cells start to reach area and start the healing process. Fibroplasia cells coordinate the replacement of defective cells with new cells and begin the healing process.

CONNECTION OF AGE-RELATED CHRONIC DISEASES AND INFLAMMATION

Research in the last decade has shown that there is an association between chronic inflammation diseases and the development of heart disease, diabetes, Alzheimer's, various cancers and aging.

INFLAMMATORY FACTORS

$\Rightarrow$ Infections, as colds, flu, parasites, etc.
$\Rightarrow$ Trauma and physical injuries, burns, fractures, cuts.
$\Rightarrow$ Aging, the breakdown of tissues that occurs throughout life.

⇒ Environmental factors, air pollution, smoking, ionizing radiation, sun burns and strenuous exercise.
⇒ Food allergies, celiac disease, lactose intolerance, poor diet and nutritional deficiencies.
⇒ Free radicals

DIAGNOSIS OF INFLAMMATORY CONDITIONS

⇒ Abnormal white blood cells in blood count
⇒ Elevated sedimentation rate of erythrocyte
⇒ Elevated levels of CRP

NUTRITIONAL THERAPY FOR INFLAMMATIONS

Food can affect your levels of inflammation. Researcher Monica Reinagel published a book called The Inflammation Free Diet Plan. She lists an index of hundreds of food inflammation levels.

Here are some foods to give you an indication of how the levels look. the higher the number the effects are positive and helps inflammation. The lower the number the less effective the food is. the minus numbers aggravate the inflammation.

FOOD INDEX – ANTI-INFLAMMATION

⇒ Natural salmon, 100g = 493
⇒ Tuna in oil, 1 can, inflammation level = 275
⇒ Cooked broccoli, ½ cup, inflammation level = 73
⇒ Olive oil, 1 tbsp., inflammation level = 73
⇒ Almonds not roasted, 30g, inflammation level = 56
⇒ Cauliflower, 1 cup, inflammation level = 18
⇒ Cherry tomatoes, 1 cup, inflammation level = 14
⇒ Lean meat, 200g, inflammation level = 10

FOOD INDEX – PROMOTING INFLAMMATION

⇒ Cooked lentils, ½ cup = -6

⇒ Apple, 1 medium, inflammation level = -30

⇒ Whole wheat bread, 1 slice, inflammation level = -31

⇒ Walnuts, 30g, inflammation level = -38

⇒ Butter, 1 tbsp., inflammation level = -45

⇒ Hardboiled egg, No.1 small, inflammation level = -51

⇒ Chocolate ice cream, ½ cup, inflammation level = -127

⇒ Cornflakes, amount 1 cup, inflammation level = -182

⇒ French fries,1 portion, small, inflammation level = -336

AVOID

⇒ Foods containing Arachidonic acid

⇒ Fried foods and barbecue cooked foods

⇒ Foods with a high glycaemic index

⇒ Foods containing Trans fats

⇒ High consumption of dairy products

⇒ Foods containing lectins

NUTRITION

⇒ Whole foods, preferably vegetarian diet

⇒ Foods with a low glycaemic index

⇒ Foods containing omega 3

⇒ Vegetables and fruits in all colours

⇒ Nuts and seeds

⇒ Olive oil

⇒ Spices and herbs rich in antioxidants

⇒ Oats rich in GLA

⇒ Drink plenty of water

SUPPLEMENTS THAT CAN HELP

⇒ GLA – fatty acid
⇒ Omega 3
⇒ Celadrin
⇒ Turmeric
⇒ Quercetin complex
⇒ Grape seed extract
⇒ Vitamin D

Chapter 14

What IS Health?

Premise to help your body heal and strengthen itself.

How can you define what is health? How do you know you are healthy? You usually establish your general physical health by there being an absence of symptoms of disease, pain or disability and all your bodily functions seem to work without disturbances.

You live a relatively healthy lifestyle without too much exposure to second-hand smoke, toxins or too much pollution. Your emotional health is generally judged by your ability to function in society within normal acceptable social behaviour, and you can support yourselves and function seemingly well in a daily routine.

So basically, if there is nothing to indicate otherwise you can assume that you are healthy. Not trying to scare anybody, but how do you really know you are healthy? Conventional medicine doesn't investigate further if your blood tests don't show anything out of the ordinary. You have all sorts of screenings like mammograms, ultrasounds or MRI's that show that you don't have symptoms of any disease.

But showing that you don't have a disease does not mean you are in optimal health. A lot of times your blood tests show acceptable results, which means that you are healthy now. But if you look at what the results are indicating toward if you continue your current eating habits and lifestyle, you anticipate preventable health issues. You are then able to avert these problems from arising by making the necessary adjustments to your nutrition and lifestyle, and work toward optimal health.

Being in optimal health, first, is what prevents a lack of health, which then helps prevent diseases from developing. In the holistic world, you check your life force. It is a triangle of three life sustaining elements that function freely and without blockage. Being healthy enough is not optimal health especially when it is in your power to change the situation around.

LIFE FORCE IS ALWAYS SET TO HEAL

By NUTRITION

Nutrients to maintain optimal health

By MOTION

Systems in your body are constantly in motion keeping you alive

By DRAINAGE

Execretion of toxins and waste products keeps away disease

What can influence your health are the foods you choose to eat. Eating high quality foods that are rich with vitamins and minerals replenish and nourish your body. The food you eat is what is fuelling your body with energy, the nutrients are transported in your blood stream providing the much-needed energy into your body, so you can stay healthy.

An indication of your health is how you feel. Your energy level is your vitality, healthy skin, and clear eyes, healthy shiny hair, feeling happy and optimistic. It is a holistic belief that prevention is the best medicine. Rather invest in your health when you are healthy by buying healthy food and eating well than the other way around. Investing in your health now ensures that your body will have all the right tools to assist you to maintain optimal health.

STRONG LIFE FORCE	WEAK LIFE FORCE
Shining eyes	Dull eyes
Strong, steady voice	Weak voice
Erect posture	Bent posture
Full shiny hair	Dry, falling out, split hairs
Healthy complete skin	Dry itchy skin
Vital energy, high	Lack of energy, low vitality
Optimistic	Pessimistic
Happy	Sad

IMPROVING YOUR LIFE FORCE ENERGY

Strengthening, managing life force – nutrition, Bach flowers, aromatherapy oils, reflexology, food supplements, healing plants, shiatsu, energy work.

Repair body fluids and composition – nutrition, healing plants, and food supplements.

Purification and cleansing programs – fasts, healing plants, food supplements, hydrotherapy, reflexology, and more.

DIFFERENCE BETWEEN HEALTH AND DISEASE

Disease – When the number of toxins entering the body is larger than the amount going out.

Detoxification – When the evacuation of toxins is larger than the toxins entering the body.

Health – When optimal evacuation of toxins occurs then the body is more vital.

Stress is a very common term used in modern society to describe a very fast pace of life. Stress is usually the culprit in causing so many of your imbalances and deterioration to your health. So just like a good nutrition plan, it is a good idea to take time for yourself to relax and slow down and not to react to life, take control of how you live your daily life. What you feel inside can be seen outside through your external physical symptoms.

I believe that a lot of diseases you can get are preventable through healthy living. It is very possible to heal your body physically and emotionally through food. I have seen this from my own experience with my clients that I treated by simple changes to their nutrition. I know many people find it hard to believe that a simple thing like changing your diets can have such a drastic effect on your health. But you see so many times the bad effects that unhealthy food has on people.

Think of how many times you yourselves have had a negative reaction to food, and you all know of someone suffering from heart disease because of a bad diet. It really is then logical to assume that if unhealthy foods impact your body negatively so healthy nourishing food can impact your body positively.

Lifestyle affects your health, and so many diseases are preventable. Changing your nutrition and lifestyle habits, like for example, stopping smoking and start exercising regularly can add years to your life. Diseases are not fun, or cool, and it is certainly no fun suffering from a horrible disease like emphysema at age thirty-eight because you smoked like a chimney since age eleven. These days thirty-eight years old is young.

At this age a lot of people are looking ahead at their future. Having to deal with a problem like emphysema which is an old person's disease at 38 would be very frustrating, being young with an uncool old and debilitating disease.

If you can prevent or lessen your chances of getting emphysema, heart disease, or diabetes and more by simply eating healthy and living a healthy lifestyle, then why not. If you know that your family has a history of heart disease, wouldn't and shouldn't you like to learn more about healthy living? Being healthy is the goal always. When you are healthy you have so many opportunities and possibilities open to us.

Consider all the life sustaining functions that your body must do just to keep you alive even before you do anything strenuous such as get out of bed in the morning. While you were sleeping, your heart was pumping blood into your body. Your lungs were cleansing the toxic blood that was pumped in from the heart, and with breathing in oxygen could supply the heart back with the clean oxygen rich blood filled with nutrients to deliver into your body.

Our liver was filtering toxins by producing bile to absorb all the poisons. Your brain is responsible for your involuntary nervous system that gives orders to the heart, lungs, liver and all the other organs to perform their tasks. This is just a small part of what your body does while you not aware of it. To be able to keep this up it takes energy, which your body gets from the food you eat. This is called your BMR, your basal metabolic rate, which is the number of calories you need to maintain your life.

Doing the responsible thing is to support your body, feed it with nutritious food, and keep your body weight at a normal range. This would also allow your hearts to work easier and help prevent heart disease. Eating fast food is very offensive to your liver and gallbladder which work very hard filtering toxins, salts and fats from your blood stream. As you know there are huge amounts of toxins, salts and fats in fast foods.

Drinking plenty of water or herbal tea with no sugar is great to assist your kidneys to flush out. Your pancreas deals with all the sugar. I believe eating a cookie here and there is okay, but it would be better if they were homemade.

Manufactured food is always full of unnecessary preservatives, colourings and margarine. I always say, "know what you are eating." If you would like to eat cake, and maybe have the time, it is so much better to bake it at home using healthier and purer ingredients. It is sad that it is so hard to find natural foods in the shops these days.

Eating the wrong foods has been made too easy for you by the large food chain companies, making it more convenient for you to buy rather than cook. With your busy schedules, it is much easier to buy a hamburger instead of preparing yourselves a sandwich. For some of you this has become so normal that you don't even realize that what you are eating is so unhealthy.

The truth is that it is hard to understand unless you see for yourselves the chemicals and types of ingredients used to make the food look like what it is supposed to resemble –

hydrogenated junk food like potato chips or all those things that come in those plastic bags. As you can see, I don't know too much about them. I have not touched them for years. I suggest that you all do the same. These are pure poison. There is nothing even chemically close to food in any of those products.

A poor diet always has a negative impact on your health, if not immediately then later, always causing deficiencies and diseases. It is important to make that extra effort to give your body foods that are rich with vitamins and minerals so that it has the necessary tools available to it to maintain your optimal health.

I know that if you don't have any serious diseases it is easy to say next time, I will be careful. I also understand that you cannot go a lifetime without eating chocolate or cookies or whatever, so really try to moderate. Since the cells in your bodies are just two days old, eating healthy food gives your body the proper tools to rebuild itself. Whatever you ate the day before yesterday is what your cells used to renew themselves, and that is what you are made up of today

.

Chapter 15

Understanding Nutrition

Why do you need a nutrition plan designed for you?

Nutrition is nourishment. Food filled with nutrients replenishes your body allowing it to function optimally. Your body uses nutrients to fuel and supply all your cells via the blood stream to enable them to rejuvenate. This is really what you are made of. If you eat junk, then your body is filled with junk. Food also affects the way you smell; bad body odour can be an indication of the food you have been eating.

Meal planning is very important for your digestion to ensure that you eat regularly so that you don't go for long periods of time without eating and replenishing your body, and it lessens the craving for junk food.

THERE ARE SIX MAJOR NUTRIENTS

⇒ WATER

⇒ CARBOHYDRATES

⇒ FATS

⇒ PROTEINS

⇒ MINERALS

⇒ VITAMINS

Water – It is important to drink plenty of water. It was once thought that an average person needs at least eight glasses, but I think it is very individual. So please drink, even if you don't feel thirsty. Non-caffeinated teas, without sugar, are also a great way to hydrate yourself. Eating a lot of vegetables is also a nice solution. There is a lot of water in vegetables, so this is an extra form of hydration. It is important to keep your urine clear to protect your kidneys, keeping them functioning normally.

Carbohydrates – are formed in plants during a process called photosynthesis that produces the glucose, which is carbon dioxide and water combined with solar energy. Carbohydrates are found in all parts of the plant but are mainly produced from the roots and seeds that contain the starch. Carbohydrates are then accumulated in the form of glycogen and stored in the liver, muscles and kidneys and are released slowly when needed as an energy source.

A good source of carbohydrate is from whole grains, beans, potatoes, legumes and root vegetables, pasta, rice or bread. Whole grains release their sugars into your blood stream at a much slower rate than a bar of chocolate. this prevents your insulin levels from shooting up and then crashing down at a dangerous rate. Eating carbohydrates that have extra fibre in them, like whole grains, oat bran, or wheat bran also prevents you from being constipated, so eat plenty of whole grains and vegetables.

Fats – are classified as saturated or unsaturated depending on their structure of fatty acids. Saturated fats generally come from animal fats, and unsaturated fats generally come from vegetables. Beware of trans-fats, guys, they are very rare in nature, and have been shown to be highly detrimental to human health, but have properties useful in the food processing industry, such as rancidity resistance – which basically means it doesn't decompose naturally only chemically.

Essential fats- as human beings you need at least two fatty acids that are essential and must be included in your diet.

Omega-3 ALA alpha-linolenic acid is derived from linolenic acid which is then converted into eicosapentaenoic acid EPA, and docosahexaenoic acid DHA, by your body. ALA can be found in many vegetables, beans, nuts, seeds, and fruits.

Omega-6 fats are derived from linoleic acid and are found in leafy vegetables, seeds, nuts, grains, and vegetable oils corn, safflower, soybean, cottonseed, sesame, sunflower seeds.

Omega-6 fatty acid, gamma-linolenic acid GLA, has been shown to have anti-inflammatory effects and fights disease GLA can be found in rare oils such as black currant, borage, and hemp oils.

So be sure to eat health oils, such as, walnuts, almonds, olive oil and avocados to name but a few. Just remember you don't need to eat these in large quantities.

Protein –your body requires amino acids to produce new proteins, especially protein retention – such as muscle mass, and to replace damaged proteins, like damaged muscles. As there is no protein or amino acid storage provision, amino acids must be part of your diet.

If you eat too much protein, then amino acids are discarded in your urine. Therefore, if you constantly eat too much protein it causes stress in your kidneys. About 20 amino acids are found in the human body, and about ten of these are essential and, therefore, must be included in your diet. How much protein a person needs depends on your gender, amount of activity you do, your weight and your height, and needs to be calculated individually for your daily caloric intake.

It is possible to combine two incomplete protein sources for example, rice and beans, to make a complete protein source, and characteristic combinations are the basis of distinct cultural cooking traditions. However, complementary sources of protein don't need to be eaten at the same meal to be used together by the body.

Sources of dietary protein include meats, tofu and other soy products, eggs, legumes, and dairy products such as milk and cheese. Excess amino acids from protein can be converted into glucose and used for fuel through a process called gluconeogenesis. the amino acids remaining after this conversion are discarded.

Minerals – dietary minerals are the chemical elements required by living organisms, other than the four elements carbon, hydrogen, nitrogen, and oxygen that are present in nearly all organic molecules.

Minerals are essential nutrients that your body needs in small amounts to function properly. Minerals can be found in varying amounts in a variety of foods such as meat, cereals and bakery products, like bread, fish, milk and dairy products, vegetables, fruits and nuts. Vital minerals have three main functions, building strong bones and teeth, regulating cellular metabolism, and transferring the food you eat into energy.

VITAL MINERALS

⇒ Calcium
⇒ Iron
⇒ Magnesium

⇒ Phosphorus

⇒ Potassium

⇒ Sodium

⇒ Sulphur

Vitamins – Fat-soluble vitamins, which include A, D, E, and K, are stored in the liver and used up by the body very slowly. Because the body stores fat-soluble vitamins, they can be dangerous when taken in large amounts. Water-soluble vitamins include vitamin C and the B vitamins. The body uses these vitamins very quickly. Excess amounts are removed in the urine. As with the minerals discussed above, some vitamins are recognized as essential nutrients, necessary in the diet for good health.

WHAT IS A NUTRITION PLAN?

A nutrition plan is a healthy eating plan that gives your body the nutrients it needs every day, either for weight loss or to maintain your weight. Based on natural foods a nutrition plan helps train your taste buds to like the taste of natural foods, seasoned with very little or even no salt or sugar. When you can come off sugars and simple carbohydrates like white bread, white sugar, etc., you can get used to a whole new world of food.

A nutritionist will design a nutrition plan for you which takes into consideration your age, gender, height and weight. The amount of exercise you do and how active you are in your daily life. The nutritionist works out how many calories you need and of those calories how much will be from fat, carbohydrates or proteins. This is the basis of a balanced daily diet based on healthy foods especially for you.

This is not so simple, and a lot of time is spent on designing your specific plan. Taken into consideration are allergies, or maybe you are vegetarian, vegan or just don't like certain foods or if you need to lose or gain weight. These preferences will all be part of your personal nutrition plan.

The advantage of eating natural food is that you will look and feel so much better when your addiction to sugar weakens. Resisting the urge eat junk food and processed food that the food industry which is a big weakness in your society is always tempting you to buy. Junk food gives your body's metabolism a hard time detoxing. You crave sugar and monosodium glutamate and all the other addictive preservatives that processed foods contains. You have become unaccustomed to eating vegetables and don't like them.

If you look at natural food, you see that it is a real blessing to feast your eyes on the miraculous variety of colours, sizes and textures of real food. When you start living and nourishing yourselves on natural food such as fruits, vegetables, legumes, whole grains, essential fats and more, as food sources you feel more alive and vibrant. You use all your senses when you buy natural food...that you are not able enjoy from purchasing processed foods.

You love to touch and smell the scent of a lemon, a honeydew melon has such an alluring aroma, and you love the shape and its freshness. To go with this amazing world of natural food is the amazing world of spices and herbs, for example baking sweet potatoes with rosemary is a great way to enjoy a vegetable that you would usually not touch.

Fill your home with fresh herbs of all varieties. If you are able to, you can maybe grow a few plants on your windowsill like mint, sage, oregano and lemongrass to name just a few. Discover spices and chilies – use them to help you to start loving natural foods.

Chapter 16

The healing properties of Vegetables

Incorporating Them Into your Daily Diet

Vegetables are what you are usually too lazy to eat. I don't know why it seems such an effort to eat them, yes even for me. Maybe you just need to change your outlook towards vegetables and see them as fun and exciting. Vegetables when served well are very pleasing to you and stimulate all your senses. They are very aesthetic, they also add colour and variety to your plate, and once you are exposed to their natural taste, they are very palatable.

As you will see vegetables comes in such a wide variety of shapes and colours, and really are so good for us. Vegetables being a major supplier of your vitamins, minerals and water. Their healing properties are profound, and you are constantly learning more about their qualities and how much they enhance your health and beauty. Learning more about vegetables and how to eat them, you will start understanding which vegetables are better for you and your own personal digestive tract.

It is now 2017, and because of so much social media exposure there is really no excuse of not being aware, you all know now that vegetables are good for us. But now it's time to make the effort to understand why they are good for us. It is time you stop viewing a plate of vegetables as a punishment and give them credit for all the great things they do for us. Not just for your health, but also your beauty and quality of life.

The World Cancer Research Fund recommends consuming large quantities of vegetables because they contain antioxidants and fibre that may help prevent cancer. They advise you to consume vegetables of all kinds and a wide spectrum of colours and parts of the plant to consume a variety of nutrients.

Many case studies of the effect's vegetables have on older people, found that vegetable intake can slow the aging process and reduce the risk of developing heart disease and blood vessels. Being rich in cellulose and minerals like iron, calcium and potassium, and they are low in sodium.

You will learn that green vegetables are rich in vitamin C, and beta- carotene are found in orange vegetables and so on. Once you understand why Vitamin C is good for us, you will make the effort to eat the right vegetables (or fruits). It is always preferable to get your essential nutrients from natural sources and less from a bottle. When you eat food, your bodies digest the food by breaking it down stripping the vitamins and minerals from the food.

Your body then transfers all the different nutrients to which ever organ is responsible for its storage. Vitamins are either fat soluble or water soluble. Fat soluble vitamins A, E, D & K, are stored in the liver and your fat tissue. Water soluble vitamins B & C pass right through your body, so these are important to replenish daily. In this way, your body transfers the food you eat into your very own DNA.

Vegetable you eat should be fresh as possible and must be stored in the refrigerator. When you cook vegetables in water, you should try and keep their cooking to a minimum. Prolonged cooking and reheating destroy their flavour and vitamins, especially of water-soluble vitamins like C and B. Over cooking also destroys a large part their other nutritional values and mineral cortex. Because vegetables are sprayed with so much pesticides which penetrates the soil and roots, it may be advisable to consider either not to eat the vegetables in their peels or eat organic vegetables.

Chapter 17

Red Vegetables
Contain lycopene Bioflavonoid.

Lycopene is a bright red pigmentation that gives it its flushed colour in your liver and blood. Lycopene originates from the carotenoid family and is now gaining recognition as a source of protection from certain diseases, such as cancer and heart disease because of its antioxidant effect.

Lycopene is a very strong antioxidant and its strength is very long lasting. It tends to accumulate in the body and affects prostate health and sperm production. Tomato consumption reduces cancer in these organs. Tomato and lycopene have been in the spotlight since studies have shown that increased consumption of tomato products was associated with a significant reduction in the risk of prostate cancer.

A diet rich in tomatoes contributes to maintaining the health of your heart and blood vessels, approximately two a day is recommended. Lycopene in Tomatoes is attributed for its ability to act against oxidation processes. Two of tomato every day during the week could also help in lowering cholesterol levels in your blood.

The yellowish gel that surrounds tomato seeds are aspirin like component, they reduce the risk of blood clots. Studies demonstrate the ability of tomatoes to prevent against blood clots forming.

Tomato and lycopene also maintain eye health and may also help in maintaining normal vision. It was recently discovered that high concentrations of lycopene in parts of the eye, producing the watery fluid that fills the eyeball. Lycopene protects and helps your eyes to re-focus on objects. As a result, lycopene protects against two problems Glaucoma - which can lead to blindness and aging when you start to find it difficult to focus on small objects.

Tomato and lycopene protect you from sun damage a new German study found that consumption of tomato paste for10 weeks protected skin from reddening when exposed to the sun. Participants in the study were exposed to UV radiation and at the same time were treated with tomatoes. Authors concluded following this study and following further studies that lycopene and other carotenoids can serve as protection from sun damage and thus contribute to skin health.

> ⇒ Lycopene levels is much higher in red tomatoes than in paler or green tomatoes.
> ⇒ Lycopene found in red tomatoes, watermelon, papaya, pink grapefruit and guava.
> ⇒ Lycopene is insoluble in water and is fat-soluble, so it is best to eat fresh or cooked tomatoes with a small amount of oil like olive oil.

Cooking tomato solidifies its cellular structure and increases the availability of lycopene and its rate of absorption. It is recommended to eat well cooked tomatoes and other tomato products, in addition to fresh tomatoes.

Facts about Lycopene

⇒ Vitamin c
⇒ Antioxidant
⇒ Vitamin K
⇒ Essential for blood clotting
⇒ Vitamin B 6
⇒ Essential for the metabolism of protein
⇒ Iron
⇒ Prevents anaemia, and assists in normal functioning of the brain and learning ability
⇒ Potassium
⇒ Tomatoes contains fibers that enable the operation of the digestive tract

Red Vegetables - Chinese Nutrition

Summer-Dew-Red-South-Bitter

Fire   Yin Qi

Actions   downwards, drainage

Organ   heart

Functions   anti-inflammatory drains moisture and heat

Bitter food – coffee, green tea, rye Beet, Dandelion Root, Okra, Red Bell Pepper, Scallion, Tomato

Bitter sour – olives, vinegar

Bitter Spicy – green onion, turmeric, orange peels, radish leaves

Bittersweet – asparagus, celery, lettuce, quinoa

An easy way to remember this is that red foods are red like blood and improve circulation.

SOME EXAMPLES OF RED VEGETABLES

Red Pepper - contains a large amounts of beta carotene and potassium. Beta-carotene is a pro- vitamin which means that it is a substance that may be converted within the body into Vitamin A. Beta-carotene actively encourages and facilitates enzymes and has the ability to inhibit enzymes associated with DNA synthesis of cholesterol by reducing blood cholesterol levels in your body. Vitamin A and beta-carotene also contribute in assisting your immune function, normal growth in children and the maintenance of healthy skin.

Absorption of beta-carotene is enhanced if eaten with fats as carotenes are fat soluble. Such as a pumpkin eaten with pumpkin seeds, ready made by nature. Red pepper is also one of the seven vegetables that contains lutein which is one antioxidant for blue light absorption in the eye, having an important role in maintaining eye health. Lutein is essential for preventing macular degeneration in the eye and protecting the lens of the eye from cataracts.

Red pepper is also a good source of vitamin C, it contains more than five times the amount of vitamin C than a navel orange. A medium sized pepper contains a respectable 230 mg.

Hot red pepper - Hot pepper is one of the oldest domesticated crops in the Western Hemisphere and is the most widely grown spice in the world. Hot red pepper contains a phytochemical called Capsicum which is also a powerful antioxidant as well acts as an anti-inflammatory. Capsicum is found in nature to have antifungal and antibacterial properties, acting as a deterrent to animal predation.

Hot red peppers reduce the risk of cancer by causing the increasing and accelerating of body heat, this inhibits the substitution rate of cancer cells thus inhibiting the growths of several forms of cancers. Ingredients until half an hour after eating the pepper. Causing a burning sensation

Hot pepper has been used as a medicine for many generations. Scientific studies indicate that Capsicum is real contributor in the reduction of the risk of the vascular inflammatory process. Hot pepper is used to treat diseases cardiovascular system and blood vessels. In Herbal medicine, it is used to stimulate circulation, by massaging the skin by being added to a base oil, never directly on your skin. Hot red pepper is used as a remedy for rheumatic pains and arthritis and has an aesthetic effect well the ability to distracting you from localized pain.

Another great virtue of hot red pepper is the ability for it to reduce your appetites and help promote weight loss.

Chapter 18

Yellow/Orange Vegetables

The Carotenoids family.

These are a large family of very lightly pigmented minerals that give many fruits and vegetables their color. Carotenoids are known for their bright orange colour, although their colours range from pale yellow to bright orange and deep red which is directly linked to their structure. Xanthophyll are often yellow are also known as Lutein which is synthesized only by plants.

Like other xanthophyll's they are found in high quantities in green leafy vegetables such as spinach, kale and yellow carrots. There are currently 600 recognized carotenoids which are divided into two main groups, the carotenoids and the xanthophyll.

Carotenoids may also slow down the aging process and reduce complications associated with diabetes and improve lung function. They also reduce the risk of heart disease, stroke, blindness and various types of cancer.

All carotenoids are built from carbon and hydrogen and some carotenoids contain oxygen atoms. The un-oxygenated carotenoids such as a-carotene, beta-carotene, and lycopene, are known as carotenes. Carotenes name derived from carrots, these are carotenoids and Carotenes typically contain carbon and hydrogen only. Carotenoids with molecules containing oxygen, such as lutein and zeaxanthin, are known as xanthophyll.

Carotenoids and chlorophylls are the major pigments involved in light harvesting and energy transfer process in the natural photovoltaic synthesis. Carotenoids does this by consuming light at different wavelengths than lights engulfed by the chlorophylls. Carotenoids are an antioxidant that neutralizes free radicals, therefore plants rich in carotenoids are able to help prevent cancer. Not all the carotenoids become retinol, and to do so they require body fat and a number of minerals, the main one being zinc. Zinc assists the carotene in its ability to transfer from carotene to retinol.

Zinc is a mineral of great importance because of its role in tuning and regulating your bodily processes. Zinc assists your body to integrate vitamins and produce insulin and Beta –carotene. Beta-Carotene is a cancer fighter; it improves communication between cells. It does this by activating genes which produces tiny openings in the cell, this allows the transfer of information from cell to cell.

Abnormal cell communication may be one reason the uncontrolled cell growths, leading ultimately to cancer. Lycopene and lutein also help communication between cells, however, beta-carotene but does it best.

A simple tip, when frying in oil put a piece of carrot into the frying pan, this retains the oil's quality by neutralizing any free radicals generated during the frying process.

Carotene you now know are known for their natural antioxidant properties and great for inflammatory bowel disease, ulcers, and Crohn's colitis. Do not eat vegetables rich in cellulose raw, it is best to cook the vegetables because cooking softens the cellulose and enables easier digestion. Some examples of vegetables containing beta-carotene are, carrots, sweet potatoes and pumpkin.

Carotenoids and retinol are accumulated mainly in the liver and fat cells, liver reserve supplies finish quickly when the body is busy healing a disease and helps your immune system cope. Disease conditions that interfere with normal digestion and absorption leads to pancreatic and liver diseases and frequent gastroenteritis can therefore impede the efficient absorption of retinol and carotenoids. Smokers and people on very low dietary fat diets tend to have low levels of carotenoids and are high risk for these diseases.

Beta-carotene helps control enzyme activity associated with the production of cholesterol. Also, other components such as the dietary fibre in carrots contribute to the reduction of cholesterol levels. The consumption of two large carrots a day for a week reduces levels of Cholesterol by as much as 10%. Research studies have also found that increased carrot consumption contributes to reducing the risk of stroke.

The federal government's 2010 Dietary Guidelines for Americans notes that nutrients should come primarily from foods. Intact Nutrient-dense foods contain not only the essential vitamins and minerals that are often contained in nutrient supplements, but also dietary fibre and other naturally occurring substances that may have positive health effects. In certain cases, fortified foods and dietary supplements may be useful in providing one or more nutrients that otherwise might be consumed in less than recommended amounts.

Facts about Beta-Carotene

⇒ Beta-Carotene is a natural antioxidant
⇒ Bright orange in color
⇒ They are Fat Soluble
⇒ Provitamin A carotenoid
⇒ It takes 12 mcg of beta-carotene to make 1 mcg of retinol
⇒ A deficiency is treated by eating more foods high in vitamin A

Yellow/Orange – Chinese Nutrition

Earth - centre incense - yellow - up and down - Sweet

Actions	Raises
Earth	Yang action
Organ	Spleen, Stomach
Functions	Harmonizes, relaxes, soothes, feeds via fluids, moisturizes, strengthens energy, builds up yin

Sweet foods – 80% of foods are considered sweets: carrots, sweet potatoes, pumpkin, beetroot, fruits, rice, wheat, and oats

Some Examples Yellow/Orange Vegetables

Carrots - carrot contains yellow orange pigmentation called beta carotene which gets it source colour from the carotenoid's family. Pro vitamin A is a significant and vital vitamin proven for maintaining the proper functioning of your immune system. It also ensures normal growth, maintenance of healthy skin and the reduction of cancer risks.

Carrot contains beta-carotene, a source from Vitamin A, fibre K, vitamin E and vitamin C. Carrots also contain good source Minerals, the main one among them is potassium that contributes to the reduction of heart disease. Carrots also contain folic acid and B-complex. Can keep blood pressure down, reduce the risk of certain cancers, such as mouth cancer and prostate cancer.

Carrot juice is considered useful to fight anaemia and help with atherosclerosis, asthma, cholesterol, congestion, constipation, ulcers and water retention. Carrot Juice assist the liver to excrete bile and excess cholesterol. Carrots relaxes the intestinal wall and protects the nervous system. Carrot juice helps protect the skin from sun damage and acne. There tends to be a high concentration of pesticides in carrots, so chop approximately one cm from the top and bottom edge or consider buying organic carrots.

Carrot Juice has great benefits for nursing mothers as it can help them enrich their milk. It can also help supply calcium during pregnancy. Carrot juice is also an excellent way to ensure that your breastfeeding infant receives adequate vitamin A.

Per Chinese medicine carrots strengthens blood and beneficial anaemia, it is because amber is considered in Chinese medicine strengthens spleen

Carrot juice is not recommended for diabetics.

Excessive consumption of carrots can color your hands and feet in orange, this phenomenon is not harmful.

Sweet potatoes - Sweet potato contains large amounts of beta-carotene, and is very rich in calcium, potassium and fibre. Sweet potatoes are also rich in vitamin C and is a reputable base as a staple food with vitamins and minerals.

Sweet potatoes and its juice segment are very effective for facial skin. The Juice together with the pulp smashed are very effective for easing arthritis.

Per folk medicine it is recommended as a first food for babies after weaning from breast milk. Additionally, per Chinese medicine, sweet potato will benefit even to those trying to lose weight, because the natural sweetness of the sweet potato strengthens the spleen. The spleen is responsible by the Chinese on the mechanism of hunger and satiety, so strengthening the spleen lead to satiety and decrease the need for sweets,

Strengthening the spleen strengthens the blood vessels, so the potato - very suitable for people who suffer bruises hematomas resulting from a small blow.

Chinese medicine also say, sweet potato is the most balanced food, orange colour and how its growth Connectors her element earth. Potato warm and very suitable for adding winter dishes.

Pumpkin - By Chinese medicine as pumpkin as an orange food, strengthens parts - spleen, causing the effect of satiety, metabolism improvement materials, strengthening the immune system and preventing mucus. Another claim to the Chinese that the natural sweetness of the pumpkin allows the body to get a sweet taste extent, and thereby reduce the need for dessert others. It heats and appropriate supplement to any dish a winter like soup and stews. Folk medicine say pumpkin contributes to strengthening the hair roots and is suitable for skin and hair dry.

Pumpkin oil is great for skin and dry hair, grate pumpkin coarsely, put in jar pulverized with a glass quart capacity, add a mixture of these oils.

⇒ 30mls Jojoba oil
⇒ 30mls Grape seed oil
⇒ 60mls Almond oil.

Completely cover the pumpkin, save the oil well and add a tablespoon of wheat germ. Seal the jar and place on a windowsill lit and warm place for two weeks. Every day shake the jar, after two filters the oil in a dark bottle through cheesecloth and squeeze the garlic well, seal and store in a dark place, the oil remained two years.

Use the hair once a week before shampooing Spread the scalp and massage well, aside for half an hour, preferably in a towel oil staining overlapping the head. - Usage skin once a week after cleansing face spread the oil min 20 - and massage the face and neck, suspend the current input Spread cream.

Chapter 19

Green Vegetables
Contain lutein Green.

Greens and plants due zeaxanthin blood called chlorophyll green plants; chlorophyll is essential for photosynthesis in the plant to produce oxygen. In addition to the plant produces chlorophyll and carotenoids lutein antioxidants to protect itself from the harmful effects of free radicals generated when sunlight strikes chlorophyll. As the darker green plant also contains more chlorophyll and need more antioxidant protection, so plants green and dark between them constitute a particularly rich source Lutein

FACTS ABOUT LUTEIN

⟹ Lutein comes from the word luteus meaning yellow.

⟹ Lutein is synthesized only by plants and like other xanthophyll is found in high quantities in green leafy vegetables, lettuce, spinach, parsley, chard, dark green zucchini and yellow carrots.

⟹ Lutein is also rich in natural antioxidant and for blue light absorption.

You accumulate Lutein in or retina, eyes and serves as a photo protection against free radicals' effects on your retina that are produced by blue light. Clinical trials have demonstrated a benefit for lutein in macular degeneration in a study, in which the researchers concluded that visual function is improved with lutein.

Lutein maintains eye health and is one of the main antioxidants in the eye, it plays an important role in the prevention of macular degeneration, which is a major cause of blindness in adults. The disease is caused by the degeneration of the macula, the most sensitive area of the retina. Macular degeneration causes the centre field of view of the person to disappear.

Researchers from the Howard study in 1994 posted in a ground-breaking finding that people who ate foods with carotenoids, drastically reduced their risk of macular degeneration. A low risk was also found among subjects who ate two vegetables containing high lutein. Spinach as well as collard greens have found to have an association between lutein and macular degeneration.

Lutein absorbs blue light, which is most damaging to the macula, the blue light causes the formation of free radicals that damages over time the light-sensitive cells that allow you to see. Wearing sunglasses with yellowish or brown lenses can filter and alienate part of the harmful light-absorbing rays, however, the rest of rays need eye benefit from a dietary lutein intake. It is very important because your body cannot produce Lutein on its own.

There are 3 main high-risk groups for whom it is important to ensure that they absorb Lutein.

⇒ Women because their eyes don't produce high quality lutein as efficiently as men.

⇒ People with blue eyes, because their iris is light and allows more light to enter the eye, which is harmful to the back of the eye.

⇒ People with a family history of macular degeneration.

Lutein is also found in the lens of the eye and protects against cataracts. Light enters the eye passing through the lens. Over a lifetime, your lens proteins are harmed by sun exposure and damage by free radicals, showing evidence of burdening cellulose generated under the influence of UV light. The light hardens the cataracts and eye develops a murky eyesight.

EXAMPLES OF YOUR GREENS

Avocados are rich in so many nutrients such as Vitamin K, Folate, Vitamin C, Potassium, Vitamin B5, Vitamin B6, Vitamin E, Magnesium, Manganese, Copper, Iron, Zinc, Phosphorous, Vitamin A, B1 Thiamine, B2 Riboflavin and B3 Niacin.

Broccoli contains a lot of vitamin D, there is a large deficiency epidemic in the world. When large supplemental doses of vitamin D are needed to offset deficiency, ample supplies of vitamin K and vitamin A help keep your vitamin D metabolism in balance. Broccoli has an unusually strong combination of both vitamin A and vitamin K.

GREEN VEGETABLES ACCORDING TO CHINESE NUTRITION

Spring - Wind – east- Sour

Actions   contraction, inward contraction

Wood   Yin Qi

Organ   Liver

Functions   collects, ties, and cools, prevents leakages, centres, neutralizes toxins, lacks mental stability, good for bleeding, too much sweating, diarrhoea, and haemorrhoids

Sour food – vinegar, lemon, apple vinegar, apple cider

Bitter sour – olives, vinegar

Sweet sour – peaches, loquat, Chinese orange, apricots, pineapple

Spicy sour – leek

People with a tendency to eat sweets after meals should eat sour to neutralize the urge.

Chapter 20

Blue/Purple Vegetables

Contain anthocyanin and appears red, purple or blue.

They belong to the flavonoid molecule class and are synthesized via the phenylalanine which are organic compounds that are synthesized by plants from the amino acids. They are found in purple cabbage, eggplant and are odourless and nearly flavourless, contributing to taste as a moderately astringent sensation.

In photosynthetic tissues such as leaves and sometimes stems, anthocyanin have been shown to act as a "sunscreen", protecting cells from high-light damage by absorbing blue-green and ultraviolet light, thereby protecting the tissues from high-light stress.

FACTS ABOUT ANTHOCYANIN

⇒ Anthocyanins comes from the Greek word Anthos meaning "flower" and also from the words kyaneos/kyanous that means "dark blue".

⇒ Anthocyanin are water soluble vacuole pigments that give a red, blue or purple colour and even may appear blue or black, depending on their PH level.

⇒ They are present in all plant and fungal cells and belong to the flavonoid family. Food plants rich in anthocyanins include the blueberry, raspberry, black rice, and black soybean, among many others that are red, blue, purple, or black.

Some of the colors of autumn leaves are derived from anthocyanins and occur in all tissues of high growing plants, including their leaves, stems, roots, flowers, and fruits of the plants. Anthocyanins has a protective role in plants against extreme temperatures countering reactive oxygen leading to a lower rate of cell death in leaves.

INTRODUCING YOUR BLUE/PURPLE VEGETABLES

Purple cabbage contains one of the highest levels of vitamins and minerals. Raw purple cabbage gives you many reasons to consume this vegetable. A single serving of raw purple cabbage contains about 20 percent of your daily requirement of vitamin A, it also contains vitamin C. Other vitamins and minerals include folate and vitamin K; calcium; magnesium; and potassium.

Egg Plant, Aubergines are a spongy, absorbent fruit from Australia and New Zealand. It is a plant species in the nightshade family and contains Solanaceae. Many plants of this family contain potent alkaloids, and some are highly toxic, but many of them, such as, tomatoes, potatoes, eggplant, bell and chili peppers are used in our daily cuisine. Aubergines absorbs oils and flavors into its flesh through cooking that makes it popular in Middle Eastern kitchens.

Raspberries contains phytochemicals one of which is anthocyanin pigments. Raspberries got their name because they were known as raspise "a sweet rose-colored wine". They are a rich source of Vitamin C, Manganese, Vitamin A, thiamine, riboflavin, vitamin B6, calcium, zinc and dietary fiber.

PURPLE VEGETABLES – CHINESE NUTRITION
Winter Sunshine - black – north - Salty

Actions	downwards and inwards
Organ	Bladder, Kidneys
Water	Yang Qi
Functions	Annexes fluids, softens lumps and hardenings, encourages excretion and neutralizes toxins
Salty food barley	seaweed, miso, salt, sardines, soya sauce,

Chapter 21

White vegetables
Contain sulphuric compounds.

Most of us never think white when thinking about vegetables. We usually think of all the other colors, however when we think about it look how many white nutrient rich vegetables are available to us. Onions, garlic, onions, leeks, cauliflower, and kohlrabi, potatoes, turnips, parsnips, mushrooms. White vegetables contribute substantial quantities of nutrients that you seem to be missing most often like potassium, magnesium, and fibre.

FACTS ABOUT SULPHURIC COMPOUNDS

⇒ Sulphur is an essential element for all life and is almost always in the form of metal sulphide.

⇒ It is a chemical compound whose atoms form cyclic octatonic molecules. Elemental sulphur is actually a bright yellow crystalline solid when at room temperature.

⇒ Sulfur is the tenth most common element by mass in the universe, and the fifth most common on Earth and was known in ancient times, being mentioned for its uses in ancient India, ancient Greece, China, and Egypt.

We may recognise Sulfur from literature classes, where it was called brimstone, meaning "burning stone". Sulfur is also use for the treatment of acne and other skin conditions. It's keratolytic agent kills bacteria, fungi, scabies mites, and other skin parasites.

Potassium is a silvery-white metal that is soft enough to be cut with a knife with little force. It is also a mineral and an electrolyte ion which are vital for the functioning of all living cells for normal nerve transmissions. It helps your muscles work, including the muscles that control your heartbeat and breathing. Having a deficiency or excess of Potassium can result in some of these signs and symptoms, that may include an abnormal heart rhythm and various electrocardiographic abnormalities.

Magnesium is a shiny grey solid which has a physical resemblance to the other five elements in the world. It is the ninth most abundant element in the universe but is eighth most abundant element in the Earth. However, in the human body it is the eleventh most abundant element and is essential to all cells and some 300 enzymes. Magnesium is used in medicine for laxatives, antacids and to stabilize abnormal nerve excitation or blood vessel spasm, such as eclampsia.

Some White Vegetables

Cauliflower - Move over kale... this veggie has been deemed one of the hottest trends of the year. Along with the other members of the cruciferous family, like broccoli, cauliflower, cabbage, and Brussels sprouts, cauliflower contains sulphur compounds that are associated with fighting cancer, strengthening bone tissue, and maintaining healthy blood vessels.

Garlic - Aside from tasting great, garlic has been known as being able to help hair grow, cause acne to disappear, and keep colds and flu at bay. Its antioxidant properties can help boost your immune system and to get the most out of garlic's active chemical, allicin, cut a fresh clove up and expose it to the air for a little while before you cook with it.

Mushrooms - Get ready for this list. Mushrooms are low in calories, fat-free, cholesterol-free, gluten-free, with barely any sodium, and yet they carry a wealth of selenium, potassium, riboflavin, niacin, and vitamin D. Mushrooms are also hearty and filling so they can help you control your weight without compromising taste. And they're a rich source of umami, the fifth basic taste after sweet, salty, bitter and sour. They can help simple dishes come alive.

Onions - Chef Julia Child said, "I cannot imagine a world without onions," and for good reason. The anti-inflammatory chemical in onions, called quercetin, can help ease discomfort from arthritis, and quercetin beneficial properties have been associated with a lower risk of cancer, heart disease, diabetes, and a stronger immune system.

WHITE VEGETABLES -CHINESE NUTRITION

Fall Sounds - white – west -Pungent

Actions	Raises up and to the sides, spreads out
Organ	Lungs
Function	excretes pathogens, dries, excretes and prevents moisture. Opens pores, gets rid of parasites

Hot Spicy food – onions, ginger, cinnamon, basil, fennel, coriander, garlic, wine

Cool Spicy food – mint, spearmint radish leaves

Chapter 22

Understanding Supplements

Supplements to help your body attain optimal health.

Don't worry I am not going to list every vitamin and mineral here for you, however I will list a few to give you some idea of how important supplements are to assist your body when it is going through a hard time. You don't need to take all the supplements all of the time, but there will be times in your lives that you will need to take some of them.

VITAMIN A

Vitamin A is fat soluble, meaning it is absorbed into your body through fat. Your body stores vitamin A in your liver and you have no control over how much is absorbed into your bodies and since it is very potent you do not take vitamin A anymore. Vitamin A in large dosages causes liver dysfunction because it sinks into the liver completely and is very toxic. You now take beta-Carotene whose source is vitamin A, beta-Carotene unlike vitamin A is completely harmless. Orange coloured and is used as a powerful antioxidant. The body uses beta-Carotene to produce vitamin A.

VITAMIN A SOURCES

⇒ Fish
⇒ Egg yolk
⇒ Liver

NUTRITIONAL FIBRES LOWER THE ABSORPTION OF BETA~CAROTENE

⇒ Fresh carrot only 20% is absorbed

⇒ Cooked carrot only 30% is absorbed

⇒ Carrot juiced 100% absorbed

BETA~CAROTENE IS ONLY FOUND IN VEGETATION

⇒ Green leaves

⇒ Corn, carrots

⇒ Pumpkin

⇒ Yellow fruits

⇒ Oranges

⇒ Apples

⇒ Pears

⇒ Root vegetables

⇒ Onions

⇒ White beans

⇒ Lentils, sweet

⇒ Potato

⇒ Seaweed

⇒ Nuri, seaweed

⇒ Seeds and nuts

CAROTENE IS GREAT FOR SKIN, MEMBRANE AND CELL WALLS.

Regulating genes carrying information from DNA to the ribosome, where the protein synthesis occurs in the cell, RNA_MRNA, acts as a messenger.

⇒ Growth and development of cells.

⇒ Encourages growth, bone strength, hair, fingernails, and eyes.

⇒ Helps in some cases of cancer.

Symptoms of deficiency

⇒ Night blindness, fuzzy vision, difficulty in adjusting to light, eye infections, xeropthalmia – dry eyes, absence of tears, swollen eye lids

⇒ Problematic skin, hyperkeratosis, wrinkled skin, dandruff, dry skin, itchy skin, acne, vitiligo – signs of early aging, liver stains, dull hair

⇒ Tendency to get colds, mucus infections, breathing problems, asthma, colds, pneumonia

⇒ Dysfunction or lack of reproduction development, foetus not developing properly, development and growth dysfunction

⇒ Urinary tract infections, tendency for kidney stones

⇒ Weak immune system

⇒ Shrunken testicles

⇒ Anosmia – loss of sense of smell, usually smokers

⇒ Scarlet fever, ear infections, measles, intestinal infections, uterine or ovarian infections

⇒ Pancreatic diseases

Vitamin K1 & 2

Dosage – not advised more than 500mcg per day.

Vitamin K comes in 3 forms, K1, K2, both natural and K3 is synthetic. Vitamin K is produced naturally via the intestinal flora and is responsible for flora balance. Coagulation of blood, crucial in blood clotting, without vitamin K your blood would not clot. Encourages production of osteoblast which is the synthesis of proteins necessary to connect minerals in the bone.

Vitamin K sources

⇒ Green leaves

⇒ Alpha Alpha sprouts
⇒ Kelp, seaweed
⇒ Safflower oil
⇒ Rapeseed oil
⇒ Oat flour
⇒ Dark molasses
⇒ Liver
⇒ Egg yolks
⇒ Milk, yoghurt
⇒ Fish liver and fish oils

SYMPTOMS OF DEFICIENCY

⇒ Bruising, both internally and under skin
⇒ Long term bleeding, haemophilia
⇒ Heavy period bleeding, or after birth. Women who bleed too much are administered vitamin K.

VITAMIN B – COMPLEX

Vitamin B-Complex is crucial for intestinal function, nervous system, skin health, eyes, liver, coats mucus in mouth, muscle tone, digestive system, protects nerve cells and hormonal system. Vitamin B-Complex is all water soluble, keep cooking short and don't throw the water away when cooking legumes. You can if you are cooking carbohydrates.

⇒ Vitamin B1 – thiamine "Vitamin of Joy"
⇒ Vitamin B2 – Riboflavin, this makes your urine yellow when it is well absorbed
⇒ Vitamin B3 – Niacin, lowers cholesterol, statin works better
⇒ Vitamin B5 – Phenthothenic Acid, anti-stress
⇒ Vitamin B6 – Ferredoxin, hormones, nervous system

⇒ Vitamin B12 – Cobalamin, lives in the myelin, nervous system. Prevents Alzheimer's, if you are deficient for more than a year there is irreversible damage, taken under tongue so that it bypasses the digestive tract and goes straight into the blood stream
⇒ Vitamin H – Biotin, skin, eyes
⇒ Vitamin B9 – Folic Acid, prevents damage to foetus, best taken before pregnancy, also good for sperm, important for nervous system

VITAMIN B-COMPLEX SOURCES
⇒ Liver
⇒ Wheat germ
⇒ Whole grains
⇒ Brewer's yeast
⇒ Green vegetables

SYMPTOMS OF DEFICIENCY
⇒ Red painful tongue cracked lips
⇒ Red and oily facial skin
⇒ Over stressed
⇒ Lack of energy

VITAMIN C
Vitamin C is a water-soluble vitamin, meaning that your body doesn't store it. You have to get what you need from food, including citrus fruits, broccoli, and tomatoes. You need vitamin C for the growth and repair of tissues in all parts of your body. It helps your body make collagen, an important protein used to make skin, cartilage, tendons, ligaments, and blood vessels. Vitamin C is needed for healing wounds, and for repairing and maintaining bones and teeth.

Vitamin C is an antioxidant, along with vitamin E, beta-Carotene, and many other plant-based nutrients. Antioxidants block some of the damage caused by free radicals, substances that damage DNA. The build-up of free radicals over time may contribute to the aging process and the development of health conditions such as cancer, heart disease, and arthritis.

It's rare to be seriously deficient in vitamin C, although evidence suggests that many people may have low levels of vitamin C. Smoking cigarettes lowers the amount of vitamin C in the body, so smokers are at a higher risk of deficiency.

Immunizes, increases lymphocytes, white blood cells, stabilizes antibodies levels, and neutralizes viruses, polio, herpes, hepatitis, measles, meningitis, pneumonia, aids, and much more.

VITAMIN C SOURCES
⇒ Cantaloupe
⇒ Citrus fruits and juices, such as orange and grapefruit
⇒ Kiwi fruit
⇒ Mango, papaya
⇒ Pineapple
⇒ Strawberries, raspberries, blueberries, cranberries
⇒ Watermelon
⇒ Broccoli, Brussels sprouts, cauliflower
⇒ Green and red peppers
⇒ Spinach, cabbage, turnip greens, and other leafy greens
⇒ Sweet and white potatoes
⇒ Tomatoes and tomato juice
⇒ Winter squash

⇒ Dry and splitting hair

⇒ Gingivitis, inflammation of gums and bleeding gums

⇒ Rough, dry, scaly skin

⇒ Slow healing of wounds

⇒ Bruising

⇒ Nosebleeds

⇒ Decreased immunity

⇒ Scurvy

VITAMIN D

Vitamin D, oil soluble vitamin D3 Calcipherol, is responsible for enhancing the intestinal absorption of calcium, iron, magnesium and phosphate. It is a hormone produced from cholesterol and synthesized via ultraviolet rays UVB in the skin as a photo thermic response from direct sunlight. It mineralizes bones – that is why a deficiency of vitamin D is a sign of osteoporosis.

Most people are deficient in vitamin D. It is stored in your fat cells under the skin and is released into the body from there, and the release of vitamin D is less efficient with overweight people because it gets lost in the fat. 25% of your bodies need to be exposed to the sun to absorb vitamin D, which is basically your face, hands and feet, so don't feel you need to go out half naked, here in Israel or in any other sunny country. Ten minutes a day is enough. Extra vitamin D is transferred and stored in the liver via the bloodstream, which also supplies the bones, immune system, breast and prostate cells.

VITAMIN D SOURCES

⇒ Fish

⇒ Salmon, tuna

⇒ Egg

⇒ Liver

⇒ Dairy products

⇒ Rickets in children, stress, thin bones, weak and late development of teeth, deformed leg, chest and spinal cord, long skull

⇒ Rickets in teenagers, leg pains, swelling, muscle atrophy, defective development

⇒ Rickets in adults, bone pain, soft bones, weak muscles, osteoporosis, tooth decay, constipation, weak eye muscles and weak vision

VITAMIN E

Can be taken for long periods, but advisable to take a break to prevent body reliance. Take for 3 months, take a 2-week, break, and continue to take them after.

Vitamin E is oil soluble. There are 8 types of vitamin E, 4 Tocopherols and 4 Tocotrienols. All groups are formed out of Alpha, Beta, Gama, and Delta. Vitamin E is stored and absorbed in the pancreas and bile juices.

Vitamin E is a strong antioxidant, which lowers cholesterol and triglycerides. Its production of fatty hormones prevents and fixes mutations in membranes and DNA. It supplies oxygen to cells and muscles, expands blood cells and reduces blood pressure. Vitamin E is also responsible for sexual hormones and male reproduction. It protects pregnancy, heals skin, scars and much more.

The main product is Alpha Topherol. It is the most active component amongst the Alpha Tocopherols groups, and it is also the most natural and the most effective antioxidant.

VITAMIN E SOURCES

⇒ Wheat germ oil mainly
⇒ Can also be found in avocado oil
⇒ Whole grains
⇒ Grits, barley, brown rice
⇒ Buckwheat, kasha, rye
⇒ Dark green leaves, dandelion
⇒ Sesame, nuts
⇒ Legumes
⇒ Seaweed, kelp
⇒ Eggs
⇒ Avocado and meat

SYMPTOMS OF DEFICIENCY

⇒ Damage, atrophy or oxidization of muscle cells
⇒ Damage to blood vessels
⇒ Thrombosis
⇒ Infertility in men and women
⇒ Cysts in lungs
⇒ Muscle weakness, especially eyes, strabismus, squinting or cross eyed, stiff or cramped muscles in legs at night
⇒ Sinking of fats into muscles
⇒ Reduced function of pituitary and adrenal glands
⇒ PMS, problems at menopause – hot flushes
⇒ Chronic sores on legs
⇒ Birth control pills reduce vitamin E from plasma by 20%
⇒ Cataracts
⇒ Fatigue and weakness
⇒ Stomach contractions
⇒ Skin problems, burns that don't heal, pigmentation

⇒ Bleeding and bruises

OMEGA 3

Omega-3 fatty acids, also known as n-3 fatty acids, are polyunsaturated fatty acids that are essential nutrients for health. You need omega-3 fatty acids for numerous normal body functions, such as controlling blood clotting and building cell membranes in the brain, and since your bodies cannot make omega-3 fats, you must get them through food.

Omega-3 fatty acids are also associated with many health benefits, including protection against heart disease and possibly stroke. New studies are identifying potential benefits for a wide range of conditions including cancer, inflammatory bowel disease, and other autoimmune diseases such as lupus and rheumatoid arthritis.

The three types of omega-3 fatty acids are polyunsaturated and are essential nutrients for optimal health. ALA is found in plants, EPA is obtained by eating oily fish, cod, herring, mackerel, salmon, sardines, sea weeds and found in breast milk. DHA is a crucial component of the human brain and can be synthesized from alpha-linoleic acid or obtained from breast milk or fish oils.

MAGNESIUM

Defined is a mineral, it functions as a metabolite that affects as many as 300 enzyme functions. The main ones being Gluconeogenesis which is responsible for metabolizing glucose activation of amino acids, which are proteins RNA and DNA. It also metabolizes fats that affect vitamin D – parathyroid hormone which enhances the release of calcium from the large reservoir contained in the bones.

It synthesizes Glutathione, acts as a neuromuscular transmitter, farms calcium with potassium and sodium to protect blood volume. Acts as a regulator in intra cellular secretion of insulin which is active in ATP Mg-ATP in the body, good for heart, gets absorbed into the body via the digestive tract. Magnesium is essential to all living cells

.

Chapter 23

Making Changes

A New Way of Life – Your Goal.

So now the decision is made, you are going to actively make physical and emotional changes to your life. You are going to change the way you think and alter your lifestyle. You are going to choose to think positively and take the time to relax. But where do you begin? Literally at the beginning, you start by making a list of the changes you would like to make both physically and emotionally.

PLAN OF ACTION

⇒ Decide to Lose 10 pounds, as a start.

⇒ Plan to eat healthily in the future.

⇒ Start exercising daily.

⇒ Find ways to reduce stress.

You may need to Change jobs, and maybe other changes too.

Check out gyms and studios, compare prices. You may decide to start with walking at first.

Go to your doctor and get a check-up to make sure you can work out; you will also need a doctor's note to take to the gym.

Throw out all the junk food lying around the house, remember to be strong, the decision is made, you are going to do this.

Make a shopping list of healthy food to buy at the supermarket or health food shop.

Plan your days and set out time each day for your workouts.

You take care of your physical self in the obvious ways; you keep yourselves clean and aesthetic. Now you are going to maintain your body by eating healthily, exercising and relaxing. Relaxing is really an important factor; it is literally recharging your battery. This gives you the strength, both physically and emotionally, to keep moving forward. Exercising every day, for approximately one hour is a great start to raise your fitness level.

It is not necessary to work out for longer than that. Don't become one of those people who spends hours in the gym, running on the treadmill for 2 or even 3 hours a day. This has adverse results and will cause unnecessary injuries, which is a shame because your focus is on getting healthier. Joining a gym or hiring a personal trainer is a great way to get yourselves back on track.

Having someone watching over you and keeping an eye on your progress is very motivating. This will help you and encourages you to continue working out, so it becomes part of your lifestyle.

WORK WITH A PERSONAL TRAINER
Having a personal trainer has its advantages and it is a luxury, but if you have reached rock bottom then this could save your life. You may not be able to take that first step of making changes alone, but it is important to know that there is someone professional who can help you carry the load. Especially in the beginning when you are overwhelmed and not sure how to start your new lifestyle.

The secret that a successful businessperson will tell you is that their success in achieving their goals was hiring professionals. If you run a business you need to hire an accountant and a lawyer at least, to make sure that you know the laws and tax rules. Having a professional on your side with expertise on weight loss, nutrition, workouts, or more, is a huge weight lifted off your shoulders. The advantage is that it will give you a chance to advance much quicker and with less pain than if you started alone.

You are going to have breakdowns along this journey, and if you want to be able to get up and continue and not just hold up your arms and say, "I give up," you are going to need help, knowing that there is an address should you need "emergency" help, is so important. You are not superhuman and during this transition you are going to need someone to remind you of your decision for this change of lifestyle. You will also have many questions that need to be answered. Just simply being able to ask and get your answer is great.

REASONS TO CONSIDER HIRING A PERSONAL TRAINER

A personal trainer will ensure that you are training correctly so that your muscles are proportioned to prevent compromising your skeleton's posture. Proportioned muscles also prevent sports injuries and complications to your joints and skeletal frame. It is always best to work on your problems before training on full body workouts so that your skeleton can strengthen up first.

Motivation and a specially designed workout plan for you with a target goal and focus. Many times, you will not feel motivated to go to the gym on your own, so you won't. How many times have you wandered around the gym not sure what to do? It is a great feeling knowing that you have an organized program and know exactly what you are supposed to work on that day. When you are lost, you will soon get bored, unmotivated and in a matter of days you will no longer take advantage of your gym membership, and then soon you will stop working out at all.

Your personal trainer keeps an eye on how you are working out and your progress and will not allow you to give up. Your personal trainer comes to you and you don't even have to leave your home, if you prefer working out at home then he or she will come with equipment to suit your personal needs. For example, if you will be working on core muscles, posture and spinal muscles on that day, your trainer will know what equipment to bring.

You will learn a lot from your personal trainer who can teach you how to really live a healthy lifestyle. Your trainer will give you the tools and tips to understand what healthy living all is about and can give you a program to continue with your workouts during the days you work out alone.

Only when you have had the experience of working out with a personal trainer, will you understand how amazing an experience it is. Everything is about us, all your problems are taken seriously, and you have someone's undivided attention who wants to ensure that you get the best all round treatment. Try it and you will see what I mean. Interview a few trainers and take a trial session to choose a trainer you connect with.

A NUTRITION PLAN DESIGNED JUST FOR YOU

You work hard at your workouts, so you now must learn how to eat well to nourish and replenish your body and make sure you eat a healthy diet. This includes all the crucial food groups and nutrients, essential fats, proteins and carbohydrates. If you decide to go to a nutritionist, your plan will be based on your blood test results and will combine everything you need to maintain your health and/ or to lose weight.

Nutrition really is learning about food, which makes sense since once eaten the food becomes a part of us. I very much like to know what is in my food and believe in eating food that I know what it is made of, so really home cooking is the best option. At first it may seem too hard or you may not have the time, but once you make it a factor in your life, you get used to getting in the kitchen and soon learn that it is easier than you thought.

I must say I am very lucky I have daughters who love to cook, and since I taught them how to eat healthily, they took it further and my investment works out well. They cook great meals, all healthy and nutritious. You almost always have cooked rice in the refrigerator, and since I am vegetarian, I add a salad to it with lentils or quinoa.

Once you learn more about nutrition you will then shop for food completely differently. Your shopping cart will be a complete contrast from before. You will now buy a lot of vegetables of all different colours, shapes and scents. Spices, and herbs like, parsley, rosemary, thyme, coriander, ginger and more. Spices and herbs, besides being healthy, make your food palatable without having to use too much salt.

At a restaurant if ordering salad, it is best to ask the waitress to have the salad dressing on the side. The trick to keeping weight off are those "hidden calories." A lot of times you think you are eating a healthy dish without realizing that the restaurant's salad dressing could be up to 2,000 calories alone, what a shame that is. Taking care of yourselves and asking questions is important.

You are entitled to know what ingredients were used to make a certain dish. Getting used to controlling what and how you eat will prevent unpleasant surprises like gaining weight. For example, if the food on the menu is meant to be fried, ask the waitress to have it grilled. When I go with my kids to restaurants you always share meals, I don't think you ever ordered a whole meal for one person.

The human body is not able to handle large amounts of calories at one meal, smaller portions are much healthier and easier for it to digest. Any extra calories you take in during a meal gets stored in your body as fat.

REASONS TO CONSIDER HIRING A NUTRITIONIST

A nutritionist will make sure you are getting all the nutrients to maintain your health. A lot of times when you are trying to lose weight you tend to reduce your calorie intake too much. You may also be afraid to add in essential fats because after all they are fat!!! But even fats are necessary to eat in the correct amounts. You need them for bone health.

He or she will know exactly what foods you need for a balanced diet, because it can get very confusing. There are so many essential foods and getting them all into a balanced nutrition plan is complicated. Your body needs proteins, carbohydrates, fats, vitamins, minerals and more so it is easy to become deficient in some nutrients. Especially if you have health issues with digestive problems, emotional stress or deficiencies, a nutritionist will be able to ensure that you have an optimal health plan based on your needs. For example, for stress reduction you would lower carbs to help your body reduce its levels of cortisol.

He or she will know exactly how many calories you will need. As a nutritionist, I don't make my clients count calories, but I do like to give guideline quantities so that it is easy to stick to. Knowing how much to eat really helps and you may even be surprised by how much you can eat, a lot of times you have been eating way too little. This way you will be able to tackle your weight, health and your body mass at the same time.

That you must report back to a nutritionist will prevent you cheating. Being on a nutrition plan really takes organization. On the one hand, it is great because you know what you are going to eat, and if it is prepared and ready you are less likely to lose control. On the other hand, you cannot be lazy, having a nutrition plan means that you would have to plan your meals and prepare them ahead of time. Forgetting to plan your meals for that day and going to work for a whole day with no food really should not happen.

Everyone who has been to a nutritionist always learns so much about healthy food, even if they no longer stick to a nutrition plan and have gained 100lbs. When speaking to them they sometimes know more than me. The sad thing is that even though they know how to lose weight, they are just no longer motivated. This whole process takes time, effort, determination, motivation and strength of character. You want to make this happen and never give up and never go back to the way you were.

Chapter 24

Getting Back into Shape
Stay fit, stay thin and be healthy always.

Now you are ready and eager to start your road to good health and your enthusiasm is soaring to go. That is all fantastic to hear, and it is great to keep up this momentum. If you have not worked out for a long time it is important to remember that you must listen to your body. If you feel pain during or after your workout that does not feel right for you, then don't do it.

It is very critical that you be very aware of the intensity level of your workout and it must be attuned to your body's capability. It is important to feel success and feel proud of your personal fitness achievements, at the same time ensure that the level of intensity is realistic and within the par of your fitness level.

If you are working with a trainer make sure that they are aware of any problems you may have, so they can take that into consideration when planning your workout. A trainer must be responsible and careful not to injure their clients, so please work together with them so that your workout will be effective and efficient in enhancing your health.

FITNESS PROGRAMS

Exercise programs are designed by a certified physical fitness trainer individually for you. There are many types of programs of different levels ranging from beginners to body building. A beginner's program works on all the muscle groups in the one program in order to prepare and strengthen your skeleton for muscle building, by adjusting your posture and align the proportions between muscle groups.

A lot of you have imbalances either with your posture or joints, a program must consider all issues. This ensures that you work out and strengthen their body in the correct manner. You may have an orthopaedic problem like a kyphosis, which is an outward curvature of the upper back or a lordosis, which is an inward curvature of the lower back. Most common problems are neck muscles, shoulder joints and knees. Many women have a problem with an imbalanced pelvis, and I work a lot on that in my classes.

A lot of times these problems need to be adjusted with a combination of stretches, strengthening and stabilizing workouts. When you are given a workout program without being evaluated, this can aggravate your problems and have an adverse effect on us. Addressing all issues is important. It is all too easy to be an over enthusiastic trainer and have my clients work out with a killer program, just as long as they lose weight.... this should become a way of life for us, with a permanent weight loss.

It is important to make your lifestyle change in the safest possible way. Your bodies are a work of art, when looking at a skeleton it is daunting to think that this is what is inside of us. The only thing holding your bones together are muscles, ligaments, cartilage and tendons, biomechanically designed in the most genius way. So, when your muscles atrophy because you have been sedentary and were not able to find the time to work out, you can see the damage both in your muscle mass and in your bone density. Getting back into an organized exercise regime is a great accomplishment.

If you have not worked out for a while it is important to understand that you must get into it slowly. If you build muscle mass at a too fast rate while your joints are still weak, the muscles will dislocate your joints, and possibly cause bone fractures. So please take your time and build up your progress slowly.

You need to build up bone density too. It is not possible to catch up too quickly after not working out for a long period. Especially if you have been smoking, drinking too much alcohol and have a lot of weight to lose. You want to build muscle on a solid and balanced skeleton.

If you consider yourself not a beginner but have not been working out for over a year, technically you will still need to start with a beginner program. You need guidance to progress and develop your body and build muscle mass. It is so important to work balanced and invest an equal amount of energy on each muscle group, and not develop muscle preference. This means working your pectorals and your latissimus dorsi with the same intensity and quality of work, preventing that hunched look.

An equal amount of energy on both muscle groups will ensure a proportioned body. No muscle group should ever be left out of a responsible program. Even if you have a serious knee problem and your doctors says you can work out, you work out the muscles around the knee joint very lightly with almost no weight. This method tones and strengthens the thigh muscle at a slower rate and gives the joint a chance to heal.

Working out with an exercise program also ensures prevention of injuries. The better your muscles are developed, the stronger and more protected your skeleton is. You don't have to be a body builder or to be super muscular. In my opinion, too much muscle mass has its own problems.

Most people who are very involved with body building, do it for a short period. Your body is not designed to be too muscular; all that extra muscle also needs to be maintained and supplied with oxygen and nutrients via your bloodstream. With so much muscle mass your heart is just not able to pump your blood strongly enough to reach the peripheral nerves of your body. This is the reason why a lot of times body builders will suffer from numb fingers and toes.

WEIGHT TRAINING

Weight training is working out in a gym using a combination of machines and free weights to develop and strengthen your muscles. There are several types of fitness programs, depending on your level of fitness and how many times a week you can go to the gym.

(A) PROGRAM

The first program is called an (A) program which is designed for three non-consecutive days per week workout. This workout program includes all muscle groups to be worked on the same day. The purpose of an (A) program is to balance your muscles and fix your posture and prepare your body for progress. This is a great program for people who are starting a workout regime. This program trains them physically and emotionally so that their muscles and brains start to understand that they are now in a workout routine. It also helps them build up their co-ordination between muscle groups and within the muscle fibres. This co-ordination is important to ensure you perform the exercises correctly.

This is also a perfect program for people who want to maintain their muscle mass and don't feel the need to progress to an (AB) program. An (A) program also develops muscles without the need to be at the gym too many days a week. Changing the exercises every six weeks gives your muscles a constant challenge, the exercises can also include bench and free weights.

The difference between an (A) program and an (AB) program is with the (A) program you cannot add too many exercises per muscle group because you work on the whole body at the same workout. I usually stick to two exercises per muscle group. The (AB) program divides the workout into four days a week, where you split the muscles per days, so you can add more exercises per muscle group.

EXAMPLE OF A BALANCED (A) PROGRAM
Warm Up - 7-10 Minute Brisk Walk on treadmill

Chest

Seated Bench Press – Machine (3 sets, 10 reps)

Seated Fly's Machine (3 sets, 12 reps)

Back

Lat Pull Down, Wide Grip – Machine (3 sets, 10 reps)

Seated Low Rows, Narrow Grip – Machine (3 sets, 12 reps)

Legs

Seated Knee Extensions – Machine (3 sets, 12 reps)

Seated Ham Curls – Machine (3 sets, 12 reps)

Shoulders

Seated Military Presses – Machine (3 sets, 12 reps)

Seated Reverse Fly's – Machine (3 sets, 12 reps) Biceps

Standing Bicep Curls, Weights (3 sets, 12 reps) Triceps

Standing triceps Extensions – Upper Pulley (3 sets, 12 reps)

Lower back

Prone Back Extension, Mat – arms and legs only, head stays down (3 sets, 20 reps)

Abdominals

Stomach Crunches, Mat – 30 degrees, legs 90 degrees

(3 sets, 20 reps)

20-40 minutes' aerobic workout

40 Minutes Brisk Walk

Or

40 Minutes Recliner Bike

Rest - 1-1.5 Min. between sets

(AB) PROGRAM

After approximately two months of working with an (A) program, and if your muscles have developed proportionately, you then progress to an (AB) program. This program divides up your workout so that more exercises, sets and reps can be added to your workout.

An (AB) workout is two consecutive days and a rest day, so it would look like this,

Sunday – workout (A) chest, legs, triceps and abs.

Monday – workout (B), back, shoulder biceps and lower back.

Tuesday - Rest.

Wednesday – workout (A), chest, legs, triceps and abs

Thursday – workout (B), back, shoulder, biceps and lower back.

Friday – Rest.

Rest days are when your muscles really grow, during a workout you microscopically rip your muscle fibres, and they heal growing thicker during rest days. Muscles are designed to be challenged and to be in proportion with each other and their opposite muscle groups. When the biceps contracts against a lot of weight the triceps totally relaxes, this allows the biceps to perform a full range of motion without causing damage to the triceps. The muscle that raises the weight is the same muscle that lowers it, coordinating between themselves, the muscles ensure that the motion is manoeuvred smoothly.

BODY BUILDING

Body building is the control and developing of muscle mass beyond sculpting and into complete definition. A body builder's aim is to build muscle by the causing of hypertrophy of their muscles. This procedure forces microscopic rips in the muscle fibre from the intense resistance, the result of which is a larger muscle mass. Investing in high quality work with full range of motion, slowly with complete control, working out with maximum weight to failure for between 10-15 reps, builds muscle mass most efficiently.

If you are interested in body building, be prepared to work very hard in the gym and in the kitchen, a lot of body builders cook their own meals because their nutrition and calorie intake must be so specific. Muscles are not always a gift, and not everyone is genetically blessed with the type of body that builds muscles easily. Working out with a workout program and a nutrition plan gives you the best chance of building more muscle mass. Starting with a program designed with workouts building up from 3 days a week to 4 days and so on, until you build up to a program designed for everyday workouts.

Deciding to launch into a body builder program is a real commitment, which demands a lot of discipline for workouts and nutrition. The body building regime is very strict, the workout program is designed for training every day. The nutrition plan is based on what body building stage you are at. The first stage is the bulking in which you gain a lot of muscle mass and some fat. This is done with a very specifically designed nutrition plan that ensures weight gain. The plan includes a lot of proteins, carbs and lean fats to try and build up mainly muscle mass, but the fat gain in this process is inevitable.

The second stage is the lean stage, after you have built as much muscle mass as you can, you now sculpt. The nutrition plan now consists of very lean proteins, with low fats and no carbs. The purpose of the nutrition plan at this stage is to maintain muscle mass while losing the fat.

CLEAN BULKING

If you just want to body build and are not interested in competitions, you will probably not want to bulk up the conventional way, because of the significant unwanted fat gain during the "bulking" phase. Body builders who try to increase their muscle mass without any fat gain is called clean bulking.

Dirty Bulking

"Dirty bulking" is eating a huge number of calories, without working out their exact macronutrients, carbs, fats, and proteins. Weightlifters who want to gain mass quickly most often decide to use the "dirty bulk" method.

Nutrition goes hand in hand with body building, working out hard in the gym is good but at a certain point, if you would like to obtain optimal results from the gym you need a nutrition plan. You may need to take extra protein supplements, but this is not always necessary, it is always better to opt to build naturally.

Inform your trainer if you suffer from high blood pressure, heart problems or orthopaedic injuries or anything else. Please make sure that you have a doctor's note allowing you to train in a gym before getting your membership.

HIIT – High Intensity Interval Training

HIIT, it is a system of training that is not new but has recently been re-discovered by fitness experts who did not recommend this form of training before. Physical fitness experts within the last few years noticed that exercisers who only trained in HIIT workouts lose more body & core fat, stomach fat, percentage wise when comparing the statistics with your safer workouts. In regular workouts, you work within a certain comfort zone.

To be honest with yourselves, even when you think you are working out hard and you break into a good sweat, you are still working out within a comfort zone range. In HIIT workouts the training is completely out of your comfort zone. One sure way to train out of your comfort zone is to work out in a class with a trainer who pushes you through the gruelling workout.

HIIT has come back with a vengeance but in a new form this a safer form, but the value of HIIT workouts are now through the ceiling and this new HIIT has been tried and tested in cardiology wards in hospitals here in Israel. If you are responsible and allow people who have limitations to work within them, then everyone is able to enjoy HIIT workouts. HIIT workouts involve a variety of specific exercises working in intervals using TRX bands, steps, tubes, body bars and weights, all designed to improve your speed, agility, muscle strength, joint strengthening, your burst power, coordination and cardio, all in one workout.

A complete workout does not have to be longer than 20-30 minutes. It involves a warmup of exercises that will be done during the main workout. The core of the workout will be anything from 4 minutes to 10 minutes, after which there is a cool down, which is basically more the regular range workouts. This HIIT secret is working completely beyond your comfort zone, pushing you to beyond your limits anaerobically, without the presence of oxygen, at approximately 80%, but feeling like 110% of your maximum heart rate.

You must be at the point where you are wondering how you are going to get the energy to get through this workout. Only when you are in the middle of doing this gruelling workout do you become aware of what type of energy source the HIIT workouts demand from us. Every person at their own level can reach this level and intensity for them and done responsibly the results are admirable.

You may ask, "Won't HIIT workouts cause my body to go into a catabolic state?" Great question, the answer is nope, because these workouts are short burst. If you did this type of workout for an hour, then I would say yes. So please when it comes to HIIT workouts more is not better, high intensity is better.

WHAT IS BODY SCULPTING?
What exactly is body sculpting, and what is the difference between body sculpting and working out in the gym?

Body sculpting is muscle toning or resistance training in the studio using body weight and studio equipment such as, dyna-bands, hand weights, ankle weights, over balls, fit balls, body bars, tubing bands, to name but a few. Workouts using this equipment are designed to work out your muscles in very efficient ways, taking advantage of the different variety of resistances, directions and manipulations on the muscles and the joints.

The advantage of working with studio equipment is that as well as working out your main muscle groups you can also work on smaller muscles groups and stabilizers. Playing with angles and ranges of motions you can vary the workout to isolate specific fibres of the muscles you have chosen to work with. This type of workout is really a complete body workout and there are no limitations to what you can do. It is even possible work out with 8 reps using a combination of resistances to make the workouts more difficult.

It is great to combine your workouts with the gym, body sculpt, Pilates, yoga and other studio classes. It is very important because it incorporates a wider spectrum of motions which is so important to maintain posture, flexibility and agility.

I work a lot on functional exercises, this helps my client's function in their daily lives, and this allows their bodies to cope with their lifestyle. I also like to strengthen muscles in cooperation with what they were designed to do. For example, your inner thighs are not meant to be as strong as your quads. Your quadriceps were designed to raise up your body weight, and your inner thighs are designed to adduct, close your leg at the hip joint. A muscle too strong compared to other muscles at a joint that are supposed to be stronger can cause a dislocation.

With body sculpting I can be very creative in devising whatever combination of equipment I decide to use to work out effectively in any given class. I bring the gym into the studio so to speak. These classes can be more challenging than the gym because when I teach a class, I insist on using Pilates' principles of Contrology within the demands of the exercise. This means that you are doing the exercise in good form with proper body alignment while using stabilizers and core muscles.

WHAT ARE AEROBICS?

Aerobics means "in the presence of oxygen," or literally means "living in air," which means the use of oxygen to adequately meet energy demands during exercise via aerobic metabolism. Your body recruit's energy units from your mitochondria, the powerhouse in every cell in your body. to be training aerobically is exercising for extended periods of time of 20 minutes or more at a steady pace keeping your heart rate to between 60%-80% of your maximum HR. Aerobic exercises such as, Walking, Running, Cycling, aerobic classes or Zumba classes raises your heart rate and oxygen consumption, supplying your muscles with oxygen and energy from carbohydrates, glycogen and fat during this process.

My recommendation is that you should do some sort of aerobics at least 5 days a week, between 30-60 minutes with varying levels of intensity. I am not one of those personal trainers who believes that you need to work out until you throw up, but having said that, don't get me wrong, I am a tough trainer. I like to train people to work out at about 60%-80% of their maximum heart rate. Calculate: Men, 220 minus his age, Women 226 minus her age and 60%-80% of that, for example, a man of 35 (220-35=185 and 70% of 185=129.5 heart rate).

Whatever exercise you choose to do, it is important to take precautions. Be careful not to over exercise and cause your body injuries from stress fractures or knee injuries. If you would like to take up running and are over 35 or 40 and have never ran before, you should ideally start off slowly, and not to try to run 20 miles on your first day.

Walking for an hour either on flat ground or uphill is best for your knees. At the end of the walk is a great time to do an easy jog for about 5 minutes if you want. If you have no negative reactions from your small run, then you may build up slowly. Running every day is not a good idea, in the beginning it is best to run once or twice a week at the end or in the middle of your walk. If all goes well and your body has no injures because of your short runs, then you can up your running carefully.

Good running, walking, cycling or aerobic shoes are important to ensure that you are working out at your best. Giving your joints and muscles the opportunity to work under the best conditions so you don't get injured. Making sure that you get your feet measured so that you wear the best suitable trainers for us. Taking water with you always to prevent dehydration, and wearing comfortable sports clothes, so you can work out comfortably and without restrictions of movement. If you are cycling, wearing helmets and elbow and knee protection is necessary to prevent serious injuries.

Pilates and core fitness

Pilates is named after Joseph Pilates who designed his system of exercise which combines core workouts with Contrology. Joseph Pilates was a body builder and gymnast who worked as a physical therapist during WW1 treating most of his soldiers in their beds. The patients treated by Pilates in his ward recovered well before other patients in the hospital. He then designed his

Pilates equipment which he based on his treatment of his soldiers in their hospital beds. He designed techniques to stimulate the muscles and strengthen them without competing with the joints. When muscles are strong, and the joints and bones are weak, this can cause a dislocation of the joint and the bone to break. He was also able to do the reverse, strengthen the joints without damaging weakening or injuring muscle fibres.

All of Pilates' exercises are based on Contrology, he demanded total precision and control with every one of his exercises, so that throughout the whole range of motion of the given exercise you concentrate completely and are aware of your movement through every second of the exercise. Combining control, centering, concentration, precision, breathing and efficient range of motion is Pilates' technique of performing his specially designed exercises. Based on this control his exercises include control of breathing, stabilizing core muscles and elongation.

Pilates liked to concentrate on breathing, inhaling to completely fill the lungs and to exhale to completely empty out the lungs. He liked his patients to imagine that when breathing in they would expand their ribcage to the sides, this way they would automatically completely fill up their lungs, to exhale he would ask them to engage their abdominals and pelvic floor muscles while exhaling completely. Pilates also combines muscle groups whereas in body sculpting you isolate muscle groups. There are different forms of Pilates workouts, such as mat Pilates, Pilates with small equipment where you also use equipment such as rolls, arc, over balls, Pilates ring and more and Pilates machines using specially designed equipment that he constructed based on his patients being bedridden.

AQUA/WATER AEROBICS

Water is the earth's gift to you and water naturally makes you happy, it affects your mood and gives a sensation of fun. Water appears in nature in three common states of matter, solid, liquid, and gas. Humans love to use water for many recreational purposes as well as for exercising and for sports, skiing, and ice skating or surfing. Aqua Aerobics is one of them.

Water workouts are so beneficial for strength and cardio training, flexibility, relaxation, rehabilitation, and weight management. It is probably one of the most fun types of exercise classes you can ever take.

The advantage of water aerobics is that you benefit from the healing properties of the water and you get a great work out, using and manipulating the different motions and resistances of the water. Exercises range from high-intensity exercises like kickboxing and circuit training to mind/body workouts like tai chi, which combines tai chi and shiatsu massage depending on the temperature of the water.

Athletes use water to rehabilitate after injury or to cross-train. People with arthritis or other disabilities who can't perform land exercise use water to improve fitness and range of motion and to relieve pain and stiffness.

In the water, your age or size is not an issue, you feel almost childlike in the water, and your weight does not feel cumbersome as it does on land. Because you also don't feel your size, you can perform all the exercises with almost no limitations. In regular aerobics class, large people are very self-conscious of their size and lose self-confidence when they compare themselves to other people in the class. IN the Water, there ARE No Mirrors!!! So, everyone can have fun in a water class. Water makes you happy, and to forget about the way you look for an hour is great.

You also don't need to know how to swim for Aqua classes, I have many students who don't know how to swim yet perform exercises in the water they would not have believed possible.

Seniors who rely on a walker or wheelchair on land can stand in water with the help of flotation belts and water's buoyancy and get a great workout. The water cushions stiff and painful joints or fragile bones that might be injured by the impact of land. Water is therapeutic so that it heals injuries that are too damaged to be treated on land. Using the different types of ways water contacts with the body, like pouring over the injury or impacting it and swirling, these techniques encourage the healing white blood cells to approach the injured area and start the healing process. Exercises in the water have done miracles for people.

Chapter 25

Overtraining

What is overtraining, and are you overtraining?

Overtraining is working out during your recovery time. Which is the crucial time your muscles and joints need to recover between workouts, so that your muscles can grow and develop. Overtraining is a common problem especially in weight training, but it can also be experienced by runners and other athletes.

After an intensive training session, your body must rest to advance in your strength and fitness level. This process takes two days or 48 hours for your muscles to complete their recovery, although this depends on the level of intensity and duration of exercise. Sometimes your recovery time must be longer if the intensity of your workout was higher than usual.

You risk overtraining damage if you also have other physical and psychological stress factors, such as jet lag, ongoing illness, overwork, menstruation, poor nutrition etc. Working out with any of these conditions should be at your own pace, remember that you want to enhance your body and health, overtraining just delays your ability to advance in your training.

Bodybuilders and dieters who train in intense work outs while limiting their food intake are also likely to cause overtraining damage and a serious delay in the recovery process during the rest period. This is because their calorie deficient diet caused a protein deficiency combined with their increased rate of muscle tissue breakdown. Their body is not able to rebuild because of their insufficient protein supply.

WHAT HAPPENS TO YOUR MUSCLES DURING AN INTENSE WORKOUT?

You stimulate your muscles during workouts by overloading them with heavy weights or resistance exercises, which causes trauma or small microscopic ripping of the muscles in the process of the contraction. The now ripped or damaged muscle must rest so that it can recover, it does this by activating satellite cells, which are healing cells sent to the area of the damage.

And just like any other injury your body responds by sending out healing cells, in this case the process is re-synthesizing protein cells to rebuild and repair the muscle fibres. If you don't rest, complete muscle regeneration cannot occur. Should you continue to work out with your muscles in this condition, you cause even more muscle tissue damage.

You have now reached the phase you call "over training," which is a physical and emotional reaction to working out beyond the boundaries of your recovery capacity. Persisting in excess training and inadequate rest, causes your muscle ability to decline. Mild overtraining may require several days of rest or reduced activity to fully restore your fitness. If however you continue to train despite the situation, this causes an accumulation of damage and muscle fatigue maybe even permanent damage to your muscles.

Delayed onset muscle soreness DOMS

Delayed onset muscle soreness and acute muscle soreness are unpleasant symptoms of exercise induced muscle damage, muscle soreness combined with tenderness, stiffness, dull and aching pain that bothers you during your normal daily activities. A little muscle soreness is nice after a workout, but it is not supposed to get to a DOMS situation. This is not good for your muscles because the reduced range of motion and muscle swelling makes it hard for you to move your muscles normally.

Since it causes you pain to walk normally so you walk differently, and this different walk uses other muscle fibres that are not meant for walking to do the job of the regular walking muscles. This is called compensation. Compensation muscle use is not good for long periods of time because over time it may cause skeletal damage.

Recovering from muscle soreness

When the sore muscle is painful to touch and warm or hot, then you are at risk of an inflammation or even infection. If this is the case, then please go and see your physician because you may need anti-inflammatory pills. I am not a fan of pills. It is ideal if you don't get to this situation.

Please rest until pain has completely gone before working out again. Sometimes light aerobic exercise releases muscle tension as well as gentle stretches when your body is warm.

Run water from the shower head over muscle from all angles, upward, downward and directly. Use warm water, slowly reducing temperature until cool, Not Cold.

Aromatherapy oils that may help – 1tbsp. sesame oil, 3 drops eucalyptus oil, 3 drops peppermint oil, 3 drops cajuput oil.

Chapter 26

Relaxation

What is relaxation?

Relaxation is a technique using methods, or activity that helps you relax to attain a state of calmness.

Relaxation can reduce your levels of anxiety, stress or anger. Getting rid of stress fast is so important because it is so not good for us.

Stress management decreases muscle tension lowers your blood pressure and slows your breathing and heart rate down. Deep breathing is one of the best ways to lower stress in the body. This is because when you breathe deeply, you increase your oxygen supply into your blood stream, and this naturally calms you down and relax.

Sit on a chair with your back straight and your feet firmly on the ground

Inhale through your nose for the count of 10, expanding your ribs sideways

Exhale through your mouth for the count of 10, try and empty out lungs completely

Repeat 5 times

Another thing you can do is count how many breaths you take in a minute; the average is between 10-12 breaths per minute. With the above breathing techniques try and lower the amount of breaths per minute, six would be amazing.

Stress is necessary for life because it motivates you to work hard, be creative and learn. Stress keeps you on your toes so that your natural survival instinct stays sharp to maintain your very survival. Stress becomes harmful when it overwhelms your nervous system causing it to release adrenaline into your system and activate your fight or flight mode. You all respond to stress in different ways. You could become either overwhelmed or depressed or both.

For stress that manifests itself as overwhelming, relaxation classes like yoga, Qigong, tai chi or guided meditation are great because of the deep breathing which calms the stress.

For stress that manifests itself as depression, walking is a great form of relaxation. It naturally calms, soothes and relaxes depression, because the rhythmic motion combined with the physical activity calms you down.

Joining a yoga class, going to guided meditation classes, listening to relaxing music or taking a long relaxing walk to release that tension energy. Allowing yourself to completely relax and let go of all of the unnecessary baggage you carry around and trying to focus on the good in your life. Allowing yourselves to let go and completely relax takes a huge effort. It is letting go of the control you think you have by worrying. Worrying is usually about things that may never happen. It just takes you off track and prevents you from focusing on what you should be focusing on.

Autosuggestion, prayer or self-affirmations are a great way to declare to your inner selves positive, respectful, loving, admiring confirmative traits to raise your self-confidence and teach you to think well of yourselves. You state out loud in an assertive tone of voice a list of attributes that make you feel good about yourselves.

STRETCH AND FLEXIBILITY

Stretching is just as important as exercise. Your muscles have 'fascia' which is connective tissue that surrounds the muscles, muscle groups, blood vessels and nerves. It also binds organs together, holding them in place while permitting others to slide smoothly over each other. It is made up of collagen which ideally should be translucent.

This allows your muscle fibres to slide back and forth over each other like sliding doors so that your muscles can contract and extend, so that your body continues giving you the daily luxury of being able to stand, sit, dance, and walk and so on easily, with no limitations and pain free. It is very advisable to take care of your fascia by regular stretching.

A lot of people tell me that they hate stretching because it is slow and not dynamic. They love the action they get from a spinning or kick box aerobics class. I know most people feel that they don't "benefit" from a stretch class as a workout. They feel like they are doing nothing, almost like a waste of time. But the truth is you do benefit in many more ways.

People who stretch their body are supple, agile, and strong and the chances are that you are less likely to injure yourselves when you do your spinning class. The fact is that not stretching causes your fascia to harden and become thick and inflexible. It becomes whitish then creamish and thick. This inflexibility causes difficulty for your muscles to contract and extend. Therefore, you feel stiff and find it hard to move after sitting for a long period of time. Not stretching your fascia, it gets thicker and less pliable as the years go by, causing stress on your joints and other injuries, some of which may become irreversible.

Stretching for about 10 minutes in the morning and evening when you are warmed up, either after a warm shower or light movements is ideal. Stretching does not need to be done with exercise, you may stretch while watching a movie at night or before going to work in the morning. When stretching hold the position for at least 2 minutes, remember to breathe deeply in through your nose and exhale through the mouth, as you exhale you try and extend and go deeper into the stretch.

FELDENKRAIS

In all studios, this is the most popular class, even more than Zumba. I have seen people who could not move their joints feel much better after a Feldenkrais class. I am a big fan of functional exercises; Feldenkrais is a master at these. I used to recommend Feldenkrais mainly for older people, now I think everyone would benefit from experiencing these classes.

Young people are less agile and in general move less than you did at their age. They work hard and long hours and spend less of their time on leisure. If you are alive you will need to sit, stand, lay down and will also need to get up and out of bed. Most of Feldenkrais's classes are seated or laying down, so everybody can participate in these classes.

Great idea if you suffer from chronic pain, the Feldenkrais method reduces pain, assists you in improving your physical function, and makes you aware of yourself and your body. Feldenkrais teaches you how to move your body in many different and specific ways while enhancing your range of motion.

Feldenkrais teaches a lot of functional movements using methods like the Alexander technique to increase function with greater ease and pleasure of movement. Feldenkrais is perfect for treating specific injuries caused by habitual and repetitive motions, or by physical dysfunctions. I call it, rehabilitation by movement awareness techniques.

TAI CHI

Tai Chi is a soft martial art, or I would say even a holistic form of martial arts, with kata type forms that are performed in slow motion with control and specific movements, allowing the moves to be very deliberate. Tai Chi is done every morning in China at the workplace, employers have workers do tai Chi forms before their shift begins because of proven results that the body will have more energy after a workout.

Tai Chi works on balance, control and coordination. The katas are performed in a meditative state, using specific breathing techniques and movement awareness that focuses the mind solely on the movements of the form helping to bring about a state of mental calm and clarity.

GUIDED MEDITATION

Guided meditation is a great way to relax completely when in a class with a teacher guiding us. It is important to make sure you come prepared for this class. You need to wear very comfortable clothing, and you may like a sheet or a blanket to cover yourselves. Some people bring pillows too, whatever you need to make the experience amazing is advisable.

A meditation class can be for 45 minutes, where 25 minutes is spent on stretching and relaxation and the last 20 minutes is guided meditation.

Try it yourself, start by laying on your back with your arms at your side and go through a system of relaxation in stages, until you are completely relaxed. Take a journey to a place where you feel safe. Or take a journey inside your body. Play beautiful relaxing music to match the location of your safe place. Re-enforce positive thinking, tell yourself a lot of positive affirmations and personal protection statements. Enjoy the experience, it can physically change your stress level and mood drastically. You may find your face glowing with a joyfulness in your eyes, which can last for the next few days.

Doing a class like this every week gives you something unique. You learn how to let go and focus on what is important in your life. Worthwhile trying one of these classes.

YOGA

Yoga meditation is a focusing of the mind on a single object with the goal of creating the cessation of all thought. As thoughts dissipate, the mind becomes quiet, and you can be fully in the present moment, the Now. The techniques of meditation are simple and easy to learn, but the ability to keep your mind focused takes time and skill. It is important to learn to control your thoughts and you must practice a lot to really do so. The benefits of a regular meditation class are a reduction of stress, tension, anxiety and frustration, as well as improved memory, concentration, inner peace and whole-body well-being.

The main philosophy of yoga in general is simple, mind, body and spirit are all one and cannot be separated. In a yoga class, you work on your energy flow through the yoga positions. The foundation of all life and of the whole universe is the subtle life force energy. This mystical energy flows through your bodies and generates your every action, from gross physical movements to minute intrinsic muscle and joint movements. There are different types of energies and there are energy channels and chakra energy centres using various methods to increase, cultivate and direct spiritual energy.

HYDROTHERAPY, WATSU

Water is a chemical compound formula known as H_2o. It has relaxing properties – it naturally calms you down and lowers your heart rate. When frozen, it becomes ice or snow, a snowflake has a six-point symmetrical form in which no two are alike. Humans have a strong attraction to water.

You all love water. You were all developed in a sack of water. You take hot baths, long showers after which you always feel better. You love the pool and the beach because the waves of the sea are rhythmic, and its natural calming motion is very soothing to us, sometimes you listen to sounds of the sea to help you sleep. www.aqua4balance.com is a great website I found about all sorts or water therapies. They explain very simply and clearly about their different treatments and how to choose what is best for you.

Watsu is characterized by one-on-one sessions in which a practitioner or therapist gently cradles, moves, stretches, and massages a receiver in chest-deep warm water.

Watsu was originally developed by Harold Dull at Harbin Hot Springs, California in the early 1980's. Watsu combines elements of muscle stretching, joint mobilization, massage,

Shiatsu, and dance, performed in chest-deep warm water, around 35°C = 95°F. The receiver is continuously supported by a practitioner or therapist while being back floated, rhythmically cradled, moved, stretched, and massaged.

The effects of warm water, gentle touch, and numerous flowing movement techniques produce a deep state of relaxation. Watsu is now used worldwide as a form of passive aquatic therapy for physical rehabilitation of illness, injury, and disability.

Chapter 27

Real Solutions

Learning about how to move in the right direction.

For all situations, it is important to eat 6 small meals a day. This allows your body to start to get back into a routine and re-learn how to behave. The meal structure consists of 3 main meals of not more than 350-450 calories depending on your gender and size, and 3 small meals of not more than 150-250 calories. Your body needs healthy food regularly, no matter how fat you feel. You really have no choice now – this is the best way to get back on track.

I cannot stress enough how important it is to nourish your bodies with good quality food. People with a nine to five job will find it easier to regulate their meal schedule. In the old day's meals were served at specific c times.

They may have not been as sophisticated as us, but they certainly understood then that your bodies need routine. Obesity in the 1950's and 60's or even 70's was almost non-existent. It got introduced into your society together with fast convenient food and a stressful lifestyle.

Please try not to skip meals, with time you will learn and understand more why this is not productive to us. Below, I have written a very general example of a nutrition plan, but the purpose of this plan is to act as a nutrition guide. It is safe and gives a general picture of how to structure and plan your meals. This is not a plan that I am saying you should use for long term; you may wish for a more personal plan based on your blood test results. If this is the case, you will need to get a nutrition plan built especially for you by a nutritionist or a naturopath you trust.

STRESS — THE REAL SOLUTION

This is a guide to assist you in lowering your stress levels so that your bodies can start the healing process. As you have learned by now, when your body is under stress, either emotionally or physically, it releases anabolic hormones which is insulin into your blood stream at very high levels to protect itself. It does this to assist you in lowering the levels of adrenaline released into your system from the initial stress reaction.

This situation could be the status quo for months for some people, and for other people it could unfortunately stay like this even for years. The main thing is to remember that you made this decision and you are not going to give up. Persistence works.

Weight gain and sugar craving are the two main symptoms of your body being in stress mode, these cravings cause you to have no control over how your body reacts. The strong desire for sugar which your nervous system signals to your brain takes over. The nervous system uses your involuntary nerves to communicate, so you lose complete control of what you put into your mouth.

The sad thing is even if you eat nothing the results are the same, your body is in stress with high levels of insulin in your system causing and maintaining weight gain. Now, you are fighting a losing battle, you must get out of this vicious cycle.

Another thing that is happening is that when you do eat, you mainly eat what you are craving for, and that is simple carbohydrates and sugar, which reinforces the vicious cycle. Your body is losing cortisol by releasing it into your blood stream. This is the classic stress symptom. Your body is then desperate to supply you with more glucose, and it does this by craving sugars. This forces you to eat a lot of carbohydrates to feed it back into your system.

MY SUGGESTIONS

Omit from your diet carbohydrates for 10 days, please, please not longer than that. Many people tell me they have not eaten carbs in 10 years, but your body does need its carbohydrates. I will stress again your body must not live without carbs. This is a very temporary plan to give your body a chance to balance its chemistry.

Low impact exercise, like yoga, Feldenkrais, Pilates, tai chi, and stretch reduces stress, by doing these relaxing forms of exercise your body learns to breathe properly which increases your oxygen intake and excretes toxins, allowing your heart rate and blood pressure to lower.

Building up your muscle mass is also important to improve your body composition. Firstly, to recover muscle mass lost during this whole stress period, and secondly to improve your body's metabolic efficiency. Having more muscle mass keeps you thinner because your BMR, Basal Metabolic Rate burns more calories per hour.

Massage and meditation are other great options to reduce your stress level, a warm bath with aromatherapy oils.

3 drops lavender, 3 drops Melissa, 3 drops patchouli, mix them into a teaspoon of salt so they get dissolved into the

water. Oil and water don't mix so adding the oil into the salt ensures that it is dissolved.

Or another blend of aromatherapy oils are, 3 drops lavender, 3 drops Ylang Ylang, 5 drops bergamot, mix them into a teaspoon of salt so they get absorbed into the water.

After the 10 days, stick to staple foods like whole grains, legumes, lots of vegetables, proteins, low glycaemic foods.

Most staple plant foods are from either cereal such as wheat, barley, rye, maize, or rice, or starchy tubers or root vegetables such as potatoes, yams, and cassava. Other staple foods include pulses, dried legumes, and fruits. try to eat food that contains the following nutritional needs. Nutritional fibres.

SOLUBLE FIBRE

⇒ Legumes, peas, soybeans, lupines and other beans
⇒ Oats, rye, chia, and barley
⇒ Some fruits, including prunes, plums, avocados, berries, ripe bananas, and the skin of apples, quinces and pears
⇒ Vegetables such as broccoli, carrots, and Jerusalem artichokes
⇒ Root tubers and root vegetables such as sweet potatoes and onions, skins of these are sources of insoluble fibre also
⇒ Psyllium seed husks, a mucilage soluble fibre and flax seeds
⇒ Nuts, with almonds being the highest in dietary fibre

INSOLUBLE FIBRE

⇒ Whole grain foods

⇒ Wheat and corn bran

⇒ Legumes such as beans and peas

⇒ Nuts and seeds

⇒ Potato skins, Vegetables such as green beans, cauliflower, zucchini, Courgette, celery

⇒ Fruits including avocado, and unripe bananas

⇒ Skins of some fruits, including kiwifruit, grapes and tomatoes

⇒ Potassium, Cabbage, dandelion, dill, olives, parsley, potato skin, sage, watercress, almonds, blueberries, coconut, figs, peaches, prunes.

⇒ Zinc, Milk, whole grains, wheat bran and germ, pumpkin seeds

⇒ Magnesium, Egg yolk, almonds, pine nuts, walnuts, endive, mint, parsley, wintergreen.

You may need supplements like vitamin C, B-complex, especially because of B5. It may be useful to take amino acids and glutamine because of the loss of muscle mass during your stress period.

SAFE MODE – THE REAL SOLUTION

This is a man-made situation that occurs because of not eating regularly, too much dieting, or over exercising on a calorie deficient diet. There are so many diets out there enticing and promising you convincingly that their diet is the one that will work. These are the very diets that cause you to yo-yo up and down the scale, causing havoc to your body's equilibrium. While you are busy dieting or starving yourselves a lot of negative things are occurring in your body.

I will try and keep it simple. Your bodies are like machines that function on fuel, food, nutrition & nutrients, to keep you alive. While you are busy dieting and starving yourselves on very low and insufficient calories, your bodily functions must carry on at all costs. Your heart needs to pump blood, your lungs need to cleanse the body with a fresh supply of oxygen, which the heart uses to transfer to all your organs and brain, feeding them all with oxygen and nutrients.

This is your BMR, your basal metabolic rate, no matter what you burn your body needs that specific number of calories to keep you alive. The cost is your health, because to keep all your systems working your body will get the calories from somewhere else. Which is usually from your essential fibres like collagen, connective tissue or muscle mass which are proteins.

When you don't eat regularly or even starve yourselves your BMR lowers by 20% or 30% to conserve energy. But your body still needs to produce the calories to keep you alive and it will do this by what is called a "catabolic reaction," where it starts to eat itself, using mainly your muscle mass as a food source. Your BMR is rated by the amount of muscle mass you have, and since your body has been using up your supply of muscles your BMR now lowers. You now have a slower more efficient energy conserving body which has slowed your metabolic rate, and you also have a substantial loss of muscle mass. This means your body needs less calories to stay alive and survive, and this means you are more likely to get fat.

BMI means body mass index, which is a very general calculation of your fat and muscle mass ratio. Weight (kg) x Weight (kg) divided by your height (cm), for example, 60 kg x 60 kg = 3,600 divided by 164 cm = 21.8 BMI

 ⇒ Underweight BMI is less than 18
 ⇒ Normal BMI is between 18-25
 ⇒ Overweight BMI is between 25-30
 ⇒ Obese BMI is from 30 and above

It goes up showing that you have more fat and less muscle mass as your body composition changes for the worse. Not a good place to be, this causes your body to go into what you call "safe mode." Being in safe mode means any calories you eat will be stored as fat, or sugar which will be changed into fat later. No matter how many miles you run, or how little food you eat, your body is in safe mode with strong survival instincts that is part of your DNA.

So, doing a lot of aerobic exercises will not help us, it may give your body another reason to store fat. Your fat cells have sensors connected to your nervous system that affect your hunger cravings making you desire to eat as much fattening food as you can. This is the way your fat cells refill their supply of fat. You always have the same amount of fat cells. They just grow larger as you gain weight and smaller as you lose weight. When you lose weight, you don't BURN fat, the fat cell always stays. You USE the fat as energy from inside the cell which then gets smaller.

Even if you opt for liposuction it doesn't reduce your fat cells, liposuction just empties out the fat cells, which means you can still refill them and get fat again.

Studies have found that in very obese people whose fat cells have become so large, they develop more fat cells to store excess fat. This is very sad because losing weight in this situation is even harder, but you are not going to say impossible.

MY SUGGESTIONS

It is very important to teach your body to trust you again. So again 6 meals a day, 3 main meals of no more than 350-450 calories, and 3 smaller meals of no more than 150-250 calories depending on your gender and amount of exercise you do. You must be careful not to skip meals, and to plan your meals ahead so that you don't get to the point that you become too hungry and lose control.

Please stick to staple foods, like whole grains, legumes, lots of vegetables, proteins, and low glycaemic foods. Most staple plant foods are from either cereal such as wheat, barley, rye, maize, or rice, or starchy tubers or root vegetables such as potatoes, yams, and cassava. Other staple foods include pulses, dried legumes, and fruits.

When your body is in safe mode you must be determined and stubborn to get out of this cycle. Nutrition and meal planning are the most effective method of healing safe mode. It is very frustrating because you really expect to see results after working out and eating healthily for a month. The thing to remember is to never give up, even though it seems like your body is a lost cause, it is not.

Now you are nurturing your body, getting it back into a routine and allowing it to re-sync all your systems. Your rusty nervous system must get back into action and co-ordinate all your bodily functions again, allowing your body to work as it should. This healing process can take many months so be prepared for this to be a long process. You will need a Lot of patience and must be very organized and believe you can do it. Determination will get you through this.

Going to the gym and working on those machines, because you need to lower your BMI and raise your BMR. You must work very hard to raise your muscle mass to make up for all the lost mass. You should go to the gym at least twice a week, preferable three times and work on all your muscle groups equally.

Aerobics to maintain your fitness level of your heart and lungs, also to train your body to start burning calories as it trusts you more. Work out 4 or 5 days a week for about a half an hour. Make sure to eat food that has nutritional fibres, written above in stress mode suggestions.

SOLUBLE FIBRE

⇒ Legumes, peas, soybeans, lupines and other beans
⇒ Oats, rye, chia, and barley
⇒ Some fruits, including prunes, plums, avocados, berries, ripe bananas, and the skin of apples, quinces and pears
⇒ Vegetables such as broccoli, carrots, and Jerusalem artichokes
⇒ Root tubers and root vegetables such as sweet potatoes and onions, skins of these are sources of insoluble fibre also
⇒ Psyllium seed husks, a mucilage soluble fibre and flax seeds
⇒ Nuts, with almonds being the highest in dietary fibre

INSOLUBLE FIBRE

⇒ Whole grain foods
⇒ Wheat and corn bran
⇒ Legumes such as beans and peas

- ⇒ Nuts and seeds
- ⇒ Potato skins, Vegetables such as green beans, cauliflower, zucchini Courgette, celery
- ⇒ Fruits including avocado, and unripe bananas
- ⇒ Skins of some fruits, including kiwifruit, grapes and tomatoes
- ⇒ You may need supplements like vitamin C, B-Complex and omega 3.

MEDICAL PROBLEMS

Please consult with your doctor about medications and their interaction with foods or exercise. It is important to understand the effects your medications are having on you in general. Medications are a factor you need to consider, even though it is still important to eat healthy food and to exercise regularly. If your doctor gives the okay so again 6 meals a day, 3 main meals of no more than 350-450 calories, and 3 smaller meals of no more than 150-250 calories depending on your gender and amount of exercise you do. Stick to staple foods, like whole grains, legumes, lots of vegetables, proteins, and low glycaemic foods.

In general, this is a good chance to make to your lifestyle especially if you are taking medication but consulting with your physician first is a must. Any changes you make he or she must know about it, if he says it is okay then great. The chances are that he will be happy you have decided to make positive changes to your diet; however, he may be happier if you went to a nutritionist that would give you a plan based on your medication and health issues.

Go to the gym and work on the machines lightly and carefully or go to the studio and do somebody sculpt classes at least twice a week. Please tell the instructors if there are issues, they should know about before the class or workout begins. If you are taking medication for high blood pressure or have heart disease, then please consult with your physician about lifting weights. As a rule, very light weights should be used by people suffering from high blood pressure and heart disease.

Light aerobics to maintain your fitness level of your heart and lungs and to prevent heart related diseases. Please work out 3 or 4 days a week for about a half an hour.

Make sure to eat food that has nutritional fibres. You may need supplements but for those please consult with your doctor, even though supplements are natural they do interact or even affect the effectiveness of certain drugs. You must always be careful and clear when taking medication, so you must make sure to consult with your physician before making any changes to your lifestyle.

Chapter 28

Maintaining a Healthy Weight
How to eat and stay thin.

I know it's hard to believe but you really can teach your body to metabolize and use the food we're eating as an immediate energy source, and not store the food in glucose storage units that the body creates. The body creates these storage units for emergency survival that fat cells take as their energy supply to enlarge your body develops this habit after it has been abused for a long time, like if you had anorexia or bulimia, or unstable eating patterns where your body would go for long periods of time without food.

When you find yourselves in this situation, and it seems like you gain weight by just looking at food, then it is time to take yourselves into your own hands and decide that this cannot go on any longer. You decide to make serious changes to your lifestyle, but in some cases, you may already have sugar problems or be a pre-diabetic. You may also already have high pressure, but it is not too late at least you are making these changes now.

Even if you took blood tests to check your cholesterol, LDL and triglycerides and they seem okay, your doctor and your naturopath can see what diseases waiting to develop are lurking in your blood test results if you don't make the health changes right now. If you want to prevent this from happening, then I hope you make those changes before the doctor has to tell you to. Because by the time the doctor will tell you to make those crucial changes to your lifestyle it may be after damage has already begun. That would be such a shame, especially if you could have started making changes when the situation was still preventable.

Having a life comes with responsibilities. You were given a body to take care of. I believe that it is your responsibility to make sure you stay fit and healthy, just as importantly as you must keep your bodies clean and smelling nice. You should make every effort to prevent diseases, feed yourselves well and make sure you get all of your nutritional needs. Remember that you must eat regularly and not allow yourself to go hungry. Hunger pangs are a very bad sign. This is a sign that your body is in stress and will go into survival mode forcing it to start storing food instead of using it.

The big "secret"

What is the big secret to losing weight and staying thin, here is the answer, making a lifestyle change is a decision, and if you have made the decision to change your lifestyle and be thin, you must understand that your eating habits are very important. If you want to see serious changes to your body and your health, and you want to know how those "naturally skinny" people are always thin. There is almost no such thing as "naturally thin." It is refusing to give up and compromise the way you look under any circumstance.

You are constantly aware of the consequences, because being fat is not an option. There are foods you NEVER eat, such as, pastries, pasta, or anything with sugar, margarine and flour, especially when baked outside your home. All junk food and fast foods, fried food, processed foods that contain preservatives and colourings, sugared and carbonated drinks, milk shakes, iced coffees, salad dressings, saturated fats and sauces. I am sure I have forgotten something, but this is the general idea, all these foreign chemicals make you fat and keeps you fat.

This really is the big "secret," it is not easy, but the results of this huge effort are so worthwhile. Even thin people have this battle of the bulge, they may only weigh 130lbs, but they are constantly working hard to maintain their weight. They always calculate and plan what they eat and are not willing to compromise their thin figure for a piece of cake.

Imagine how you would feel after losing that annoying 20lbs. Imagine how much younger and healthier you would look and feel. Being able to be more active, alive and vibrant, you won't feel tired, depressed, lethargic or disappointed in yourselves. That feeling is amazing!

WHAT SHOULD YOU EAT?

Always staple foods, such as natural whole grains, rice, wheat, barley.

Legumes, such as quinoa, lentils, millet, oats, chickpeas and all types of beans, white and red kidney beans.

Vegetables, such as every type you can find in the supermarket of all different colours.

Protein such as meats, tofu and other soy-products, eggs, legumes, and dairy products such as milk and cheese.

Fruits, seasonal fruits, just remember that fruits contain a lot of sugar so keep it down to three fruits a day.

You also need some essential fats like walnuts, 6-8 halves, or 6-8 almonds and around one tablespoon of olive oil a day, and a tablespoon of natural tahini sauce or a half an avocado.

MEALS

For breakfast a good suggestion is oatmeal with oats milk and oat bran, or bran flakes with low fat milk.

About mid-morning, a good time for a fruit like a green apple and a couple of walnut halves, obviously not roasted.

Lunch would be your "heaviest meal" like salmon, chicken breast or eggs, with a slow release carbohydrate like whole grain rice and a salad. I am almost a vegan, so I would eat a vegan omelette or rice with quinoa and a large colourful salad dressed with olive oil and lemon juice.

Mid-afternoon meal could be another fruit which is now in season with 3 almonds.

Supper would be a lean protein of your choice, 2 slices of whole wheat bread with a lot of vegetables again.

Later if you get hungry again a rice cracker with low fat cream cheese and a vegetable.

Drink plenty of water and herbal teas, try not to drink more than 2 cups of coffee per day, if you can.

This is a very general plan, a better nutrition plan designed for you is much more advisable. There may be things that I mentioned that you cannot eat, or do not like. But I am motivating you to make the changes you have always dreamed of because the results are worth it.

Chapter 29

Holistic Relaxation

Connecting your body and soul.

Aroma is the scent, the way the oils affect you when you absorb them into your system via their aroma. Therapy is the treatment, the way the oils affect you when you absorb them into your system through your skin.

AROMATHERAPY

What is scent? Scent is a sense; you have neurons that have hair like projectors called cilia that identify the scent. Your sensors are capable of understanding and identifying the difference between thousands of smells. Even people who don't have the sense of smell, when they inhale a scent their brains are still affected by the scent in the same way as people who can smell.

Scents affects your emotions, you identify through scent feelings that are deep within us, and you also smell fear, so the right scent can help you dispel your fears, anxieties and stress. Scents can also stimulate through your senses the feeling of confidence and give you the push you need to progress and strive.

Essential oils are plant or flower-based oils that are a concentrated hydrophobic liquid containing strong aroma compound extracted by expression or cold pressed to extract their oil. Essential oils are extracted from the flower, leaves, bark or roots by distillation using steam if it is water based, and some oils are also extracted with alcohol, and are used in three different ways.

Physical, for example for reflexology or massage.

Feeling, sensory, for example if you have a headache, stomach-ache.

Emotional development, for example if you have an examination you would like to pass and are feeling very nervous about it.

MASSAGE

If you love touch, then massage is good for you. Touch is therapeutic, and it is a natural instinct you are born with. Massage is a very old healing therapy using touch to help soothe, relax, invigorate and stimulate your muscles and joints.

Manipulating the superficial and deeper layers of muscle and connective tissue using various techniques, to improve action and encourage healing. It is great for relaxation, stress release, lower blood pressure and a feeling of well-being. Primates pat and lay hands on each other, they have a social grooming ritual which is part of their everyday activity.

Massage was common in Chinese, Hindu, Egyptian, Persian, Japanese and Greek societies. When someone touches you, you feel their energy and it is very calming.

the use of aromatherapy oils like almond oil, grape seed oil, or other base oils used with essential oils combined to suit your personal health needs to provide you many therapeutic benefits.

Chapter 30

Liver Cleanse

Drink every morning for optimal health

A full liver cleanse is good to do every couple of months, and you can drink this every morning to keep your liver healthy.

1 freshly squeezed lemon juice, with 1 tbsp. of olive oil

½ cup water at room temperature the liver is the organ that has the most pressure because of its role in excreting poisons, so it is advisable to include additional supporting treatments, such as a liver cleanse. It is worth your while including this in your pre-cleanse, during the cleanse and in the months after the cleanse.

LIVER CLEANSE

⇒ ¼ mug of freshly squeezed lemon juice

⇒ 3 mugs of freshly squeezed apple juice

⇒ 1 tbsp. olive oil

⇒ 2 garlic teeth

Mix well in blender until foamy, drink morning and evening

½ hour after drinking above juice, drink hot mug of mint tea or chamomile tea

It is advisable to add thistle for support Castor oil compress

Strengthens liver and body systems

Use flannel or cotton wool doused in castor oil, cover with plastic bag and over it a hot water bottle, compress on body for 20 minutes up to one hour

Castor oil quickens the evacuation of toxins, stimulates peristaltic movement and incites the metabolism

06:00 – liver cleanse

Fruit or vegetable juice

Herbal tea

Regular water

Skin brushing

08:00 – juice

10:00 – juice with 1 tsp. psyllium

Cup of water

12:00 – fresh salad

Crushed salad, steamed vegetables

Portion of rice or millet with seaweed

Green leaves

Herbal tea

15:00 – juice with psyllium

14:30 – juice

18:00 – crushed vegetables, portion of millet, baked potatoes Vegetable Soup

Probiotic before sleep

POSSIBLE REACTIONS "MEDICAL BREAKDOWN"

⇒ Sweat, urine, stool all smells bad
⇒ Acne, spots or sores
⇒ Accelerated Heart rate
⇒ Headache, weakness, dizziness, fatigue, insomnia
⇒ Worsening of previous medical condition

If you go straight into a fast without the prep then the negative reactions will be at their worse than if you go into a fast after a prep, the negative reactions will be less

Juice fasts are stronger than fruit or vegetable fasts

To help prevent nausea then take an infusion of ginger

For headaches, you can do a lavender massage

You can make a compress of crumbled tofu and 2-3 tsp. of ginger, put on your forehead for 20-30 minutes

Chapter 31

CONCLUSION

Through this book you know what you must do.

Our relationship with food is a long and complicated one where you tend to have a love hate affair with it. For as far back as the beginning of humanity food was a necessity and an indulgence. Humans love to eat; the trouble is what you love to eat. Based on your DNA your body naturally craves fats, as you know fats are responsible for your survival, you cannot live without it.

Modern day eating habits have not changed much, but the food available to you has, and a lot. You no longer have the abundance of natural organic food, even though you are still exposed to an abundance of food, but they all come wrapped in a package.

Many people suffer from being at least 10% overweight if not more. First, it is very hard to resist sweet and savoury snacks which contain many un-natural ingredients like preservatives, colouring and taste enhancers like sweeteners or sodium. I know that from my own personal experience that when I get a craving for something to eat, I would love to choose a bar of chocolate.

The second issue is that a lot of the times you desire these snacks, are in between meals. To me this indicates that the quality of foods you are eating are not good enough. The food you are now consuming are packed with high sugar content giving you a fast sugar release. This satisfies your hunger now, but this also means that you get hungry again very fast. The solution is simple, you know what you should do, but the implementation of this concept is far from simple. Eating slow release foods that don't contain un-natural taste stimulators, eating food with no preservatives and preferably cooked at home. Eating complex carbohydrates, legumes, grains, vegetables and fruits.

A third issue is your modern-day food chain industry, they control what you choose to eat. You are bombarded with aggressive advertisements that are strategically placed, making "choosing" these products so obvious. Mass produced foods are made from the least nutritious ingredients, the main point being that the company's profit margin is healthy. You seem to have forgotten the reason for eating food, you tend to eat more for pleasure, which is fine, but you also should remember that you have a body to maintain. You are what you eat, your body uses the foods you feed it to rebuild your muscles, your organs and body systems by renewing your cells every two days.

Taking responsibility for your health is very important, in this book I have concisely put together foods you should be eating with their nutritional information. I feel it is very important for you not only to understand what your daily nutritional needs are but also how to choose the right foods. Being healthy is a decision, every day you could choose what you eat, and I would be so happy if I will be able to help towards that choice.

Chapter 32

Catching your dreams

Moving forward to achieving your personal goals

Imagine yourself one year from today, thinner and more toned. You weigh about 10lbs lighter and are looking 10 years younger. You are wearing nice clothes and have drastically reduced the stress in your life and you genuinely are healthy and happy.

If this is your goal, so make the decision to chase that dream right now. One year from now you could be living a completely different lifestyle, and really enjoying the results of your hard work to get there. Once you make that choice, don't let go for even one second. Hold on to that dream so tight, make it your focus and never forget why you want this so bad. Always remember where you came from, never forget how you felt being fat and unhealthy. Let this be a constant reminder and a motivator to never give up.

There will be easy days and there also will be hard days and there may even be impossible days, acknowledge that and be prepared for the emotional and physical battle of those hard days. Being determined to rise up to all challenges that you will face and deciding to stay strong under all circumstances is being loyal to yourself. This is what you deserve, stand up and protect yourself and give yourself another chance for a healthy life.

Learn to love yourselves unconditionally, just like you love your kids, and your friends. You are a valuable asset to society, think of how many people's lives have you touched and contributed to? Imagine what the world would have been like if you were never born. I promise you there are people walking this earth who would have been lost without you.

Every day find one thing you like and admire about yourself and validate it to yourself. Tell yourself how proud you are of your traits. Understand that you are unique. There is no one in the world like you. Even if you had an identical twin, you are still you. Know who you are and see your importance in this world. You are not here alone for a reason; your lives overlap with all sorts of people for all sorts of reasons.

You are here because you are meant to be, so enjoy being you, and be the best you that you can be and be true to yourself always.

Chapter 33

Health Questionnaire

Confidential medical information protected by law

PRINT OUT THIS FORM SO THAT YOU MAY FILL IT OUT EFFECTIVELY

Date: _____

General information:

Name		Referred by	
Address		Profession/Occupation	
Date of Birth/Age		Place of work	
Home Phone		Mobile	
Status		Country of Birth	
Email			

MAIN REASONS FOR CONSULTATION

One	
Two	
Three	

MEDICAL HISTORY:

Please mark your answers

Past	present	Health	Never
		Allergies	
		Appendectomy / grumbling appendicitis	

		Asthma / bronchitis, spastic	
		Brain stroke CVA	
		Cancer of any kind	
		Cholesterol	
		Diabetes	
		Drugs Use	
		Effect on digestion by eating a certain food	
		Epilepsy / cramping	
		Gallbladder problems	
		Gout	
		Heart Attack	
		Heart disease	
		Hemorrhoids	
		Hernia / Hernia of any kind	
		High Blood Pressure	
		Hypoglycemia	
		Kidney disease / kidney stones	
		Liver Disease / Hepatitis	
		Migraines	
		Organ transplantation	
		Problems in the blood vessels	
		Prostate problems (prostate)	
		Rheumatoid Arthritis (Rheumatic Fever)	
		STDs	
		Thyroid disease / thyroid	
		Other:	

Are you suffering from any of these symptoms?

Please mark answers

Yes	No	Health Symptoms
		Abdominal pain or dis- comfort the abdomen
		Back pain
		Bleeding or bruising marks appear easily
		Blood in sputum / phlegm
		Blood in the stool or urine / feces black
		Bloody vomit
		Breast pain, tenderness, disorders, lumps
		Breathing problems
		Change in appetite / thirst
		Change in mood, stress, depression, anxiety, etc.
		Change in weight
		Diarrhea or watery stools
		Difficulties in sexual intimacy
		Disorders of hearing / ear problems
		Disorders pulse / heart rate
		Disorders swallowing / throat
		Dizziness
		Excessive coughing, sneezing rest
		Fainting
		Fever, chills, night sweats
		Headache
		Indigestion, heartburn, flatulence
		Intolerance to heat or cold
		Pain, pressure or discomfort in the chest
		Pelvic pain / lump basin
		Problems at home / family

		Problems in the neck
		Problems walking, sitting, lying down
		Problems with urination / Change in amount of urine
		Sinus problems
		Skin problems
		Sleep Disorders
		Stops.
		Swelling or pain in joints / hands / knees
		Vaginal secretion, discomfort, bad
		Visual disturbances
		Weakness, lack of energy
		Work problems
		Other:

Family Medical History
Name, Age, Health problems if any

Relationship	Name	Age	Health	Alive/ Passed
Mother				
Father				
Partner/Spouse				
Sibling				
Sibling				
Sibling				
Child				
Child				
Child				
Child				

Hospitalizations

Please list hospitalizations in patients

Age cause of hospitalization

One	
Two	
Three	

Medications

Please list all the medication you take now or in have taken in the past month, including the dose. Please include also non-prescription medicines such as Advil, aspirin, birth control pill, vitamins, minerals, herbs, homeopathy, etc.

One		Reason for Taking	
Two		Reason for Taking	
Three		Reason for Taking	
Four		Reason for Taking	

Allergies

Please list allergies and if you are taking medication for them

One	
Two	
Three	
Four	
Five	

Additional Information

Current Weight		Desired Weight		Height	
Do you Smoke		How many a day		For how many Years	
Have you ever tried to stop smoking		How many times			
Why did you start smoking again after stopping					
Do you drink Alcohol			How many drinks		
Bowel Movements a day			Per week		
Texture: liquidy/soft/firm/hard					

Movement /exercise

Type of activity		Times a week	
HR during exercise		Level of Training (1-10)	
HR after exercise		Length of training Hours/Mins	
Number of hours of sleep on an average night			
Do you wake up in the morning refreshed or tired			

Personal preference

(Circle each answer)

Heat	Cold
Summer	winter
Drink Hot/Warm	Drink cold
Other	

What type of low impact exercises do you do?

How do you spend your leisure time?

Menstrual cycle

Age at first period		Age at Menopause	
How often do you get your period		How long does it last	
Symptoms before period			
Symptoms during period			
Mood Changes	Abdominal pain	Bloating	Breast tenderness

What personal goals would you like to achieve 3-6 months from now?

One	
Two	
Three	

Are you willing to make changes in lifestyle habits and your diet if required?

Nutrition Journal

In order for me to create a nutrition plan especially for you please take the time to fill in the diet diary below so I can get a complete picture. Please be sure to be honest with yourself and with me and write down all that you eat, even if it seems insignificant to you. The more information you give me the better I can work and be able to design for you the most suitable plan. Please also include in this diary if you are taking medications, vitamins or anything else.

The diary should be everything you eat for three day.

DAY 1

Date	Hour	Food	Drink	Medication

Day 2

Date	Hour	Food	Drink	Medication

Day 3

Date	Hour	Food	Drink	Medication

ABOUT THE AUTHOR

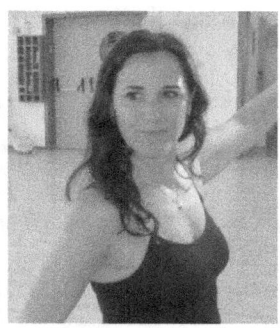

Esther Lehman lives in Israel, in Maale Adumim which is a city just outside Jerusalem, Israel. She is a personal trainer and a holistic nutritionist. She studied exercise physiology at the Wingate Institute for physical education and sports in Israel, she also studied naturopathy at the Bina Academy, Jerusalem, Israel, Esther is a black belt 4th Dan in Krav Maga. She teaches a wide range of exercise and fitness classes such as Pilates, body sculpting, aerobics, aqua, Krav Maga, and more for over 20 years.

Esther is also a massage therapist and reiki master; she believes that the body is a mirror of all thoughts. Thinking positively, with kindness and even respect, people will have a great opportunity to allow positive changes to occur in their self-perception and general health and wellbeing.

The purpose of this book to help people achieve their goals and change their life around. Ultimately the force of the changes must be generated from within you, it is easy to give up and difficult to continue the journey to success.

With success comes many failures, every successful person you know can confirm this fact.

This book is goal orientated, it gives you the tools to take charge and be in control of your nutrition and life plans.

Visit online at

https://holylandoils.com   http://estherlehman.com

I would very much appreciate it if you would take the spare a couple of minutes to write a review HERE: https://www.amazon.com/review/create-review/ref=cm_cr_dp_d_wr_but_top?ie=UTF8&channel=glance-detail&asin=1548324914#

on amazon. You might need to sign in to leave a review,

Blessings

Esther Lehman

10 Best Ways to Start Losing Weight

https://amzn.to/2yfJnsg

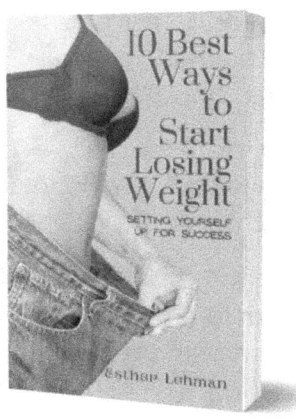

Being overweight or obese is a nightmare, and a plague for men and women of this century. You are constantly assured by others who are not overweight, that size doesn't matter, and you should all be happy with your bodies. But you know that the true reality is that size does matter.

Why are you always told its ok to be fat by thin people? Nobody likes being fat, and nobody enjoys being antagonized with fake niceties. Maybe your friends and family mean well and don't want you to feel bad or uncomfortable with your bodies, but you do.

You have many excuses for being overweight, your daily lives in this century is brutal. You are bombarded constantly with many stresses, ranging from financial to emotional. I believe that taking responsibility for your financial and emotional situations eases the path of your ability to live stress free and focus on a healthy lifestyle.

Taking responsibility for our health is of the utmost importance. In this book I have compiled the foods we should be consuming and their nutritional values. I feel it is crucial to understand what our daily nutritional needs are as well learning to choose the right foods.

Staying healthy really is a decision, every day we make these decisions when we prepare our meals. It is a privilege to take advantage of this opportunity and control what we put into our bodies.

The solution may seem so simple, we obviously know what to do... but the implementation of this concept is far from simple.

In my book you will be motivated into making the right choices of the foods you eat. We discuss the reasons for poor choices and how to avoid them. Coping with the stresses of life can cause havoc to our digestion together with what you eat regularly will affect your journey to weight loss and good health.

Plan Your Own Weight Loss Diet

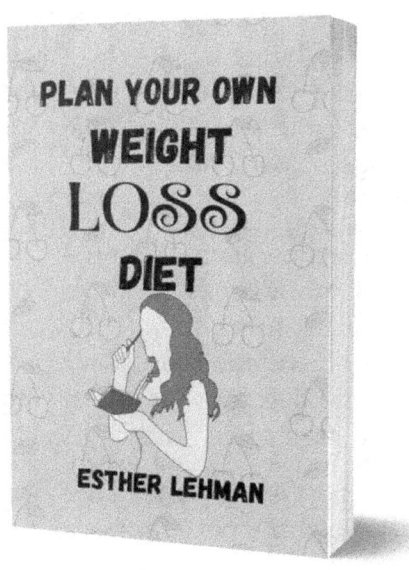

https://amzn.to/3ilV8Na

Plan Your Own Weight-Loss Diet workbook is a guide designed to make losing weight easy for you to accomplish. It is published to make your reading experience fun and exciting to use, together with your commitment to do whatever it takes to lose fat weight, we will succeed.

Go through this workbook, learn about calculating your BMI and daily Caloric needs specifically for you. Build your own Optimum Nutrition plan and start eating Smart to Achieve Healthy Living and Weight Loss.

Write down and record your progress using the specially designed worksheets, calculate the amount of protein, carbs, and fat you will need in your daily diet. You will learn how to create your own constantly changing diet and nutrition plans as you lose weight because your caloric needs will change as you will lose weight by eating right and gaining muscle.

You now have the power to make real changes to your body and health. Many times, we fear exactly the things we crave for. Our minds form a mental barrier which we must break through and focus on our goal. We must focus on our reasons and decisions for losing weight and living a healthy lifestyle, start to lose unwanted weight now.

So now the decision is made, you are going to actively make physical and emotional changes in your life. The first step is always the hardest one, but once you do, you open the channel of opportunity. We're all good at thinking big, without limitations, and really believing our dreams are ours for the taking. You can make this happen right now, buy my book, and succeed.

Ultimately the force of the changes must be generated from within you, it is easy to give up and difficult to continue the journey to success. With success comes many failures, every successful person you know can confirm this fact.

This book is goal orientated, it gives you the tools to take charge and be in control of your nutrition and life plans. I have provided many worksheets to motivate and promote action. This will make it easier for you to start to see changes happening.

Make your losing weight an easy process for you to accomplish because it is a workbook, so all the information is right in front of you to see clearly what is going on with you.

Be Accountable for Your Weight and Lose Your Fat. Taking action together with taking responsibility is accountability and taking responsibility to start losing weight by changing your eating habits. We must ask ourselves, how we arrived at this point in our lives, and this is a great place to start. Treating this journey to lose weight and drastically making changes to our lives is like a business venture.

Like in any business venture you always start by making a marketing plan. What are the first steps we must do to launch this lifestyle change? A great way is to ask our self how we got to this situation and recognizing the reasons that caused us to abuse our self with food.

Go through this workbook, learn about calculating your BMI and daily Caloric needs specifically for you. Build your own Nutrition plan and start eating Smart to Achieve Healthy Living and Weight Loss.

Write down and record your progress using the specially designed worksheets, calculate the amount of protein, carbs and fat you will need in your daily diet. You will learn how to create your own constantly changing diet and nutrition plans as you lose weight, because your caloric needs will change as you will lose weight by eating right and gaining muscle.

Essential Oils
and their Relevance to the Bible

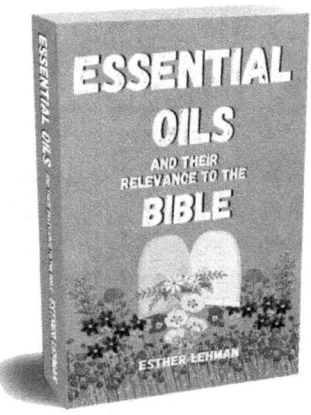

The Bible is the most read book in the world and it still fascinates readers with new and current information till today. Everything you see around you is connected to the Bible and in the cycle of life, the biblical times is not so far back. Trees that have been planted many hundred years ago are living among you with the same energy that they had in the time of the Bible.

Essential oils have been used for remedies, medications and pleasure since humans have been on earth and developed awareness. You have many beautiful trees, plants and flowers living with you and it is a privilege to enjoy them today after someone else planted them well before your lifetime. One of the most beautiful legacies you have on this earth are the amazing trees you see and take for granted. Planting long living trees such as Olive,

Pine, Cedar or Acacia is a gift for the next generations, just like the old trees you see today planted generations back for your pleasure.

Parable from the Talmud:

One day a righteous miracle worker, saw an old man planting a carob tree. Knowing that a carob tree took 70 years to bear fruit, and that therefore the old man would not live to see the results of his labour, he asked why he was planting a tree whose fruits he would never enjoy. 'Carob trees were here when I was born, planted by my father and his father,' answered the old man. 'Now I plant trees for the enjoyment of my children and their children's children.'" (Talmud Ta'anit 23a)

In Judaism it is forbidden to uproot and destroy a tree after it has been planted, you are told that you can cut them down to a stump, but their roots must stay in the ground forever. In this book I have found relevance of 108 trees and plants from around the world to the Old Testament Bible, it is amazing how much access you have today to what the people of the Bible had.

"When you besiege a city for many days to wage war against it to capture it, you shall not destroy its trees by wielding an axe against them, for you may eat from them, but you shall not cut them down. Is the tree of the field a man, to go into the siege before you?" Deuteronomy 20:19

You will learn from trees many things, like patience, strength, faith, and love.